CLINICAL APPROACHES TO TACHYARRHYTHMIAS

edited by

A. John Camm, M.D.

Volume 11

Clinical Approaches to Tachyarrhythmias (CATA)
Series Editor: A. John Camm, M.D.

CLINICAL APPROACHES TO TACHYARRHYTHMIAS

edited by

A. John Camm, M.D.

St. George's Hospital Medical School
London, United Kingdom

Volume 11

Atrial Tachycardia

by

Michael D. Lesh, M.D.

Associate Professor of Medicine
Chief, Cardiac Electrophysiology Service
Director, UCSF Atrial Arrhythmia Center
University of California San Francisco
San Francisco, California

and

Franz X. Roithinger, M.D.

Attending Physician
Department of Cardiology
University Hospital Innsbruck
Innsbruck, Austria

Futura Publishing Company, Inc.
Armonk, NY

Library of Congress Cataloging-in-Publication Data
Lesh, Michael D.
    Atrial tachycardia / by Michael D. Lesh and Franz X. Roithinger.
        p. cm.—(Clinical approaches to tachyarrhythmias ; v. 11)
    Includes bibliographical references.
    ISBN 0-87993-442-5 (alk. paper)
    1. Atrial arrhythmias. 2. Tachycardia. I. Roithinger, Franz X.
  II. Title. III. Series.
    [DNLM: 1. Tachycardia, Supraventricular—diagnosis.
  2. Electrophysiology—methods. 3. Tachycardia, Supraventricular—therapy. WG 330 C6403 1993 v. 11]
    RC685.A72L47   1999
    616.1'28—dc21
    DNLM/DLC
    for Library of Congress   99-40659
                                                      CIP

Copyright © 2000
Futura Publishing Company, Inc.

Published by
Futura Publishing Company, Inc.
135 Bedford Road
Armonk, New York, 10504-0418
LC #: 99-40659
ISBN #: 0-87993-442-5

Every effort had been made to ensure that the information in this book
is as up to date and as accurate as possible at the time of publication.
However, due to the constant developments in medicine, neither the
author, nor the editor, nor the publisher can accept any legal or any
other responsibility for any errors or omissions that may occur.

Printed in the United States of America.
This book is printed on acid-free paper.

Contents

I. Introduction

Before the modern era of invasive electrophysiology, when treatment for a regular, narrow complex tachycardia was limited to drugs such as digitalis glycosides or vasopressor infusion, the term paroxysmal atrial tachycardia (PAT) was adequate to distinguish the disorder from ventricular tachycardia. We now understand that many such tachycardias are not in truth "atrial," but may involve the atrioventricular (AV) node or an accessory AV connection. This distinction is now important, because radiofrequency catheter ablation may be offered as a curative treatment for such patients.

There is a cycle that operates in cardiac arrhythmology and electrophysiology in which the opportunity to study arrhythmias with multiple mapping catheters drives the ability to treat selected arrhythmias with specific catheter ablative techniques, which in turn requires a nomenclature that recognizes multiple, distinct arrhythmia mechanisms.[1] Such is the case with atrial tachycardias. In an era of invasive mapping and ablation, we can now distinguish between and among a number of different atrial tachycardia types, and avoid the less descriptive term "PAT."

1

In addition to invasive electrical mapping, we also have access to newer diagnostic tools such as intracardiac ultrasound imaging,[2-4] which allow us to determine the anatomic substrate for atrial arrhythmias, and body surface potential mapping,[5-7] which allows more detailed analysis of the pattern of atrial activation registered on the thorax.

Therefore, this review of the clinical manifestations of atrial tachycardia incorporates what has been recently learned from the clinical electrophysiology laboratory as far as mechanism and the potential for curative catheter ablation is concerned. By combining this perspective with more traditional methods of diagnosis and management, it is hoped that a state-of-the-art approach to atrial tachycardias will have been presented. It should be noted, however, that the study of atrial arrhythmias represents one of the fastest developing areas of clinical cardiac electrophysiology research. For example, knowledge of the relationship between atrial ectopic foci and the initiation of atrial fibrillation may revolutionize our understanding and treatment of this most common form of atrial arrhythmias. Thus, we present here our current state of knowledge, with the full realization that our understanding of mechanism and therapy will certainly evolve in the next several years.

II. Definitions

Atrial tachycardias are defined as supraventricular arrhythmias that do not require the AV node or ventricular tissue for initiation and sustenance.[8-11] This definition excludes the most common reentrant supraventricular ar-

Table 1

Classification and Definition of Atrial Tachycardia

Classification of atrial tachycardia
1) Focal atrial tachycardia
2) Inappropriate sinus tachycardia
   a) Typical atrial flutter
     i) counterclockwise atrial flutter
     ii) clockwise atrial flutter
   b) True atypical atrial flutter
   c) Incisional reentrant atrial tachycardia
3) Macroreentrant atrial tachycardia
4) Atrial fibrillation
Definition of atrial tachycardia: Exclusion of
1) Atrioventricular nodal reentrant tachycardia (AVNRT)
2) Junctional ectopic tachycardia (JET)
3) Atrioventricular reentrant tachycardia (AVRT),
  • atrioventricular
  • atriofascicular
  • nodofascicular bypass tract

rhythmias (Table 1): 1) AV nodal reentrant tachycardia, where the reentrant circuit is considered to be confined to the compact AV node or its extensions into the atrium[12-14]; 2) junctional ectopic atrial tachycardia, a rare cause of supraventricular tachycardia within the area of the AV junction that has been found to be of automatic mechanism[15-17]; and 3) AV reentrant tachycardias involving an accessory AV bypass tract.[18,19]

Definitions and terminology for atrial tachycardias can be quite confusing.[1] A variety of features have been used to classify atrial tachycardias, such as the putative cellular mechanism, features of the surface electrocardiogram (ECG), rate of the tachycardia, the response to drugs, the presence or absence of macroscopic barriers, or the presence or absence of prior surgery. The classification schema we prefer (Table 1) has the interventional electrophysiologist in mind, as it presupposes that endocardial mapping and probably catheter ablation will be performed. This seems justified, as it is the development of techniques such as radiofrequency ablation that has generated a need for an improved classification. Atrial tachycardias can therefore be divided into the following categories:

1. *Tachycardias that arise from a focal area of atrial tissue.*

   These tachycardias may be cured with focally directed radiofrequency application (Section IV). A subclassification based on preferential anatomic locations can be helpful, such as a) "cristal" atrial tachycardia; b) atrial tachycardia of pulmonary venous origin; c) septal atrial tachycardia; or d) other focal tachycardia. Although a likely underlying cellular mechanism (reentry, automaticity, or triggered activity) may be delineated in some cases, it may be impossible to confirm the definite proof, and, more importantly, endocardial mapping and successful focal application of radiofrequency energy are independent of the suggested mechanism. Therefore, we have not attempted to further subclassify based on the putative cellular mechanism.

2. *The syndrome of inappropriate sinus tachycardia, which has certain unique features and therefore dictates a separate category (Section VIII).*

   Patients with inappropriate sinus tachycardia present with a resting heart rate of over 100 bpm or a heart rate increase to over 100 bpm with minimal exertion and a P wave morphology during tachycardia consistent with a sinus node origin. The syndrome of inappropriate sinus tachycardia is uncommon, and the underlying mechanism is still unclear.

3. *Atrial tachycardias that involve reentry with macroscopic anatomic (fixed or functional) and/or surgical barriers.*

In this category, radiofrequency lesions are curative when a protected isthmus, delineated by two such barriers, is severed such that the atrial reentrant circuit is interrupted. a) In the category of macroreentrant atrial tachycardias, typical atrial flutter is the most common arrhythmia, the macroscopic reentrant circuit and the confining anatomic barriers are reasonably well defined,[20-22] and radiofrequency catheter ablation has a high success rate.[23,24] b) A variety of macroreentrant atrial tachycardias which may have a surface ECG appearance similar to typical atrial flutter but which demonstrate variable reentrant circuits probably confined by anatomic as well as functional barriers.[25] Underlying substrate, ultimate clinical significance, and the best therapeutic approach for this atypical atrial flutter have yet to be determined. c) Incisional reentrant atrial tachycardia is a macroreentrant atrial tachycardia involving a combination of natural and surgically created (incisions, patches, conduit material) barriers in patients following reparative surgery for congenital heart disease. When approaching these tachycardias for catheter ablation, techniques are required to identify a relatively protected isthmus (Section VI).

4. *Atrial fibrillation, like flutter, likely represents a common surface ECG manifestation of several different arrhythmia mechanisms and substrates. Although maintenance of atrial fibrillation is commonly considered to be due to multiple random reentrant wavelets, recent studies suggest that in some patients an underlying rapidly firing focus is responsible for the initiation of atrial fibrillation. This new finding may be of great importance relative to ablative therapy (Section V).*

In the present classification, the term "sinus node reentry" has been avoided. Sinus node reentry has been described as an intraatrial reentrant tachycardia with abrupt onset and offset and a rate different from regular sinus rhythm.[26,27] The tachycardia origin is in the sinus node region, and the P wave morphology in multiple electrocardiographic leads and the intraatrial activation sequence are similar to those during sinus rhythm. Successful radiofrequency catheter ablation for sinus node reentry has been described.[28,29] However, there is no clear evidence that "sinus node reentry" acts differently from tachycardias located on other portions of the crista terminalis, nor is there any direct evidence that histologic sinus nodal tissue is involved. Furthermore, the sinus node is a prominent structure, extending along the crista terminalis from the high right atrium at least to the mid crista terminalis.[30,31] Attempts to modify the sinus node in cases of inappropriate sinus tachycardia have shown that extensive radiofrequency applications must be performed in order to accomplish a moderate sinus rate reduction.[32,33] This is in contrast to the reported limited radiofrequency application for what has been claimed to be sinus node reentrant tachycardia. Therefore, in the present definition, what some might term "sinus node reentry" is included in the group of "cristal" tachycardias.

Tachycardia frequency, duration, and abruptness of onset and offset may provide information about electrophysiologic mechanisms, but are generally nonspecific. For example, terms that appear in the literature include the following: "sustained tachycardias," which last longer than 30 seconds, as compared to "nonsustained tachycardias"; "paroxysmal tachycardias," which begin and end abruptly and last for minutes to hours; "nonparoxysmal tachycardias," which are only slightly faster than the baseline rhythm, may accelerate, and are frequently asymptomatic; "repetitive tachycardias," which occur as brief episodes, lasting 3 complexes to 10 seconds; "recurrent tachycardias," which occur periodically, separated by long intervals free of tachycardia; "incessant tachycardias," which occur as frequent sustained episodes, interrupted by short periods of sinus rhythm; and "continuous tachycardias," which continue without interruption for days to months.

III. Electrophysiologic Mechanisms

The clinical or electrophysiologic diagnosis of "atrial tachycardia," and even the successful treatment with radiofrequency catheter ablation, does not necessarily guarantee a specific underlying electrophysiologic mechanism.[34] For example, focal atrial tachycardia can typically be cured with focal application of radiofrequency energy, but the cellular mechanism may be microreentry, abnormal automaticity, or triggered activity. The response of an atrial tachycardia to pharmacological interventions such as administration of adenosine or verapamil can be nonspecific relative to mechanism, and the literature documents contradictory responses.[35,36] Nevertheless, clinical information, the electrocardiographic presentation, and different maneuvers in the electrophysiology laboratory allow distinction of arrhythmia mechanism in most cases (Table 2).

1. Reentry

The classic example of reentry as an underlying mechanism in atrial tachycardias is either atrial flutter[20–22] or incisional reentry, following cardiac surgery for congenital heart disease (Fig. 1).[37,38] In order to sustain a stable intraatrial reentrant tachycardia, two barriers—a central boundary and a lateral boundary—are required in order to protect the reentrant circuit and prevent "short circuiting."[39] In patients with incisional reentry, the constraining barriers consist of surgical scars, such as atriotomy sites or atrial septal patches, or a combination of artificial and natural barriers such as the crista terminalis or the tricuspid annulus. Likewise, in patients with typical atrial flutter, the barriers are anatomic structures: the tricuspid annulus acts as the anterior barrier, whereas crista terminalis and eustachian ridge act as the posterior barrier.[20–22] In humans with microreentry as a postulated underlying mechanism due to electrophysiologic and

Table 2

Clinical, Electrophysiologic, and Pharmacological
Correlates of Arrhythmia Mechanisms

	Reentry	Enhanced Automaticity	Triggered Activity
Initiation: Programmed stimulation, PACs	yes	no	yes
Constant rate pacing	no	no	yes
Cycle length dependence	rare	no	frequent
Catecholamine facilitation	sometimes	yes	yes
Warm-up phenomenon	no	yes	sometimes
Pacing: Extrastimulus termination	yes	no	no
Extrastimulus acceleration	yes	no	no
Extrastimulus reset	yes	yes	yes
Overdrive termination	yes	no	yes
Overdrive acceleration	sometimes	no	yes
Overdrive suppression	no	yes	no
Overdrive entrainment	yes	no	yes
Effect of: Vagal maneuvers	no effect	transient supp.	termination
β-blockers	no effect	transient supp.	termination
Calcium channel blockers	no effect*	no effect	termination
Adenosine	no effect*	transient supp.	termination

PACs = premature atrial complexes; supp. = suppression; * = contradictory findings

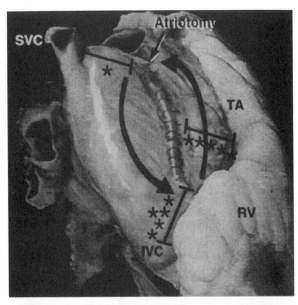

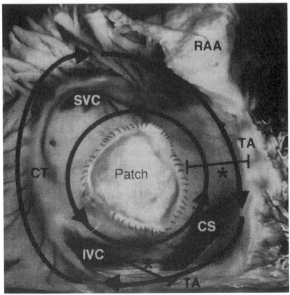

pharmacological tachycardia characteristics (Table 2), the etiology of intraatrial reentry is not fully understood.[40,41] Even in normal hearts, markedly anisotropic cell-to-cell coupling has been demonstrated for the crista terminalis in the right atrium as compared to left ventricular myocardium.[42] It may be speculated that a more rapid conduction, but with a lower safety factor for impulse propagation along the longitudinal fiber axis as compared to the transverse axis, provides the substrate for microscopic reentry.[43] It should be noted, though, that triggered automaticity and reentry might be difficult to distinguish in the electrophysiology laboratory.

Patients with reentrant atrial tachycardia are frequently older and present with a paroxysmal or constant tachycardia.[44] In the electrophysiology laboratory, reentrant atrial tachycardias are usually readily and reproducibly initiated with atrial premature beats and programmed stimulation (Fig. 2).[10,11,35,45,46] During tachycardia, premature extrastimuli may terminate and reset tachycardia, whereas overdrive pacing results in either termination or entrainment. Indeed, one can take advantage of the ability

◄—————————————————————————————

Figure 1 In patients with prior atrial surgery for congenital heart disease, natural and surgical barriers provide multiple substrates for macroreentry. Hypothetical circuits after atrial septal defect repair is shown. The epicardial aspect of the right atrium (top) and the endocardial view onto the right atrial septum (bottom) are illustrated. Both surgical barriers (patch material and atriotomy), as well as normal structures such as the crista terminalis (CT) and coronary sinus ostium (CS), can act as barriers to contain a reentrant wavefront (black circles, arrows). Bars with asterisks show relatively protected isthmuses at which ablation might be successful in eliminating one or more potential reentrant circuits. IVC = inferior vena cava; RAA = right atrial appendage; RV = right ventricle; SVC = superior vena cava; TA = tricuspid annulus. Reproduced, with permission, from Reference 37.

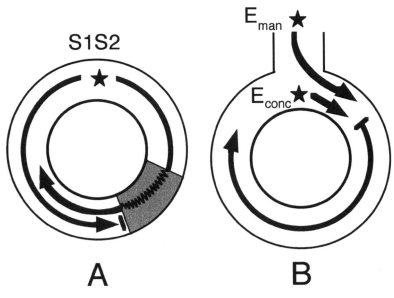

Figure 2. Schematic drawing of initiation (A) and entrainment (B) of a tachycardia with reentry as the underlying mechanism. A. Programmed stimulation with increasingly premature beats (S1S2) causes progressive slowing of conduction and finally unidirectional block (arrow with bar), possibly in an area of slow conduction (gray), which is able to induce reentry. Inner and outer circles represent the inner and outer barrier, the prerequisite for a reentrant circuit. B. Responses to entrainment maneuvers may delineate the site of pacing with respect to the reentrant circuit. During entrainment with manifest fusion (E man), pacing is able to entrain the reentrant tachycardia, but pacing is performed from outside the reentrant circuit. Surface ECG (P wave) manifest fusion is demonstrated because the atrial activation results in part from the stimulus site and in part from the last paced P wave. The postpacing interval minus tachycardia cycle length is longer than 20 milliseconds. During entrainment with concealed fusion, pacing is performed from within the narrow or critical conduction isthmus (asterisked bars, Fig. 1), and surface P wave fusion does not occur. With termination of pacing, the first P wave after the last captured P wave returns within 10 milliseconds of the tachycardia cycle length.

to terminate reentrant atrial tachycardia with pacing as a therapeutic maneuver, using transcatheter or transesophageal pacing in the proper clinical setting. Implanted devices may also take advantage of this phenomenon with their ability to detect and terminate reentrant atrial tachycardias with overdrive pacing. Vagal maneuvers, β- or calcium channel blockade, or adenosine may cause AV block, but usually have no effect on the tachycardia maintenance or cycle length.

2. Abnormal Automaticity

Abnormal impulse formation is the suggested underlying mechanism for most focal atrial tachycardias (Section IV), rapid focal atrial tachycardias initiating paroxysmal atrial fibrillation ("focal atrial fibrillation"; Section V), and inappropriate sinus tachycardia (Section VII). Frequently, the terms "focal atrial tachycardia," "automatic atrial tachycardia," and "ectopic atrial tachycardia" are used synonymously. It is assumed that a small cluster of cells demonstrating abnormal automaticity, often responsive to catecholamines, is responsible for tachycardia initiation.[35,36,47,48] Note that if the cells with a tendency toward abnormal automaticity are well coupled to the normal atrium, electrotonic interactions with the large bulk of surrounding myocardium will likely prevent these abnormal cells from firing (Fig. 3, left panel).[39] However, if the cells with abnormal automaticity are in a region of poor cell-to-cell coupling, discontinuous propagation may allow these cells to manifest their abnormal firing (Fig. 3, right panel)[49] as long as coupling is not so poor that no impulse can exit. Therefore, it may be hypothe-

Well-coupled   **poorly coupled region**

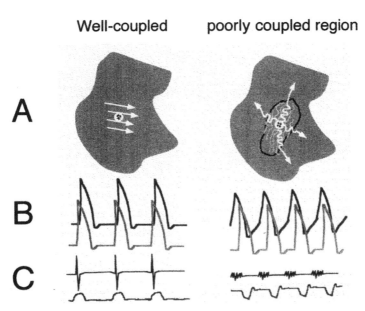

Figure 3. Illustration of the concept that regardless of the cellular mechanism of focal tachycardia, relatively poor coupling of that focus to the surrounding atrium is required to prevent electrotonic extinction of that focus. A. Drawing of atrial tissue containing a focus with a tendency toward abnormal firing. B. Simulated action potential recordings, with the black tracing from the abnormal focus and the gray tracing from the normal surrounding atrium. C. Bipolar electrogram that might be recorded from a catheter straddling the central focus and surrounding atrium, and the corresponding simulated surface P wave. A cell or small cluster of cells with a tendency toward abnormal automaticity well coupled to the surrounding normal atrium (A, left panel, gray) will not be able to manifest that tendency due to electrotonic interactions. However, if the region of abnormal automaticity is in a region of poor cell-to-cell coupling (A, right panel, black region), discontinuous propagation may allow these cells to manifest their abnormal firing. As long as the coupling is not so poor that no impulse may exit, a tachycardia can be initiated. In this case, fractionated electrograms (C, right panel) will be found during clinical electrophysiologic mapping, representing slow conduction through poorly coupled tissue, recorded from the site of the origin of tachycardia, and preceding the onset of the surface P wave by a substantial period of time, until the bulk of the normal surrounding atrium is finally activated. Reproduced, with permission, from Reference 39.

sized that abnormal cell-to-cell coupling is required in addition to an area of abnormal automaticity, if atrial tachycardia is to become manifest. Furthermore, preferential anatomic sites of tachycardia origin, such as the crista terminalis, the coronary sinus os, or the pulmonary veins, are indeed areas of relatively poor cell-to-cell coupling, either on a congenital or acquired basis.[35,50-60] The crista terminalis, for example, has been described as an area of discontinuous impulse propagation.[42]

Patients with automatic atrial tachycardia are frequently younger, have no structural heart disease (other than tachycardia-mediated cardiomyopathy, which is not uncommon), and present with a nonparoxysmal, repetitive, incessant, or continuous tachycardia.[24] In the electrophysiology laboratory, automatic atrial tachycardias are usually not inducible with programmed stimulation or overdrive pacing, but tachycardia initiation can be facilitated by administration of catecholamines.[8,35,36] At the onset, a warm-up phenomenon is characteristic for abnormal automaticity, while overdrive suppression characterizes abnormal automaticity during tachycardia and pacing. Vagal maneuvers, β-blockade, and adenosine may cause transient suppression, whereas calcium channel blockers usually have no effect.

3. Triggered Activity

The documentation of triggered activity as the underlying mechanism of atrial tachycardias has been described in rare cases,[61] and the general significance of triggered activity as an atrial tachycardia mechanism is unknown. Chen et al[35] described prominent delayed afterdepolarizations in the recordings of monophasic action potential just before the onset of atrial tachycardia, whereas recordings remote from the exit site did not demonstrate any afterdepolarization. In the electrophysiology laboratory, atrial tachycardias with underlying triggered activity are said to be inducible with constant rate pacing, sometimes facilitated by catecholamines.[62] Overdrive termination and acceleration may be observed, and vagal maneuvers, β-, and calcium channel blockade, as well as adenosine, usually terminate atrial tachycardias with underlying triggered activity. Finally, studies[63–65] suggest that paroxysmal atrial tachycardia due to digitalis intoxication is caused by triggered activity, as digitalis has been shown in in vitro studies[64] to induce delayed afterdepolarizations and triggered activity. The rapid firing of focal atrial fibrillation initiators from the pulmonary veins suggests a possible triggered mechanism.

IV. Focal Atrial Tachycardia

1. Clinical and Electrocardiographic Presentation

Patients with focal atrial tachycardia usually present with paroxysmal sustained atrial tachycardia if reentry is the underlying mechanism, but with repetitive atrial tachycardia or continuous tachycardia if it is caused by abnormal automaticity. Patients with a reentrant mechanism are older, and an underlying cardiac disease is more frequently present, as compared to automatic atrial tachycardia.[24] While atrial cardiomyopathy may be the cause of atrial tachycardia, continuous atrial tachycardia may itself cause a tachycardia-induced cardiomyopathy, especially in children, that is fully reversible after successful treatment.

The Role of P Wave Configuration

As atrial tachycardia is still a relatively uncommon form of supraventricular tachycardia, limited data are available about the value of the P wave morphology in predicting the site of origin or the mechanism of tachycardia. Tang et al[53] studied the P wave morphology in 31 patients undergoing atrial endocardial mapping and subsequent radiofrequency ablation of a single atrial focus. They found that leads aVL and V_1 were most helpful for distinguishing right atrial foci from left atrial foci: the sensitivity and specificity of using a positive or biphasic P wave in lead aVL to predict a right atrial focus were 88% and 79%, respectively. The sensitivity and specificity of a positive P wave in lead V_1 in predicting a left atrial focus were 93% and 88%, respectively. Furthermore, leads II, III, and aVF were found to be helpful for providing clues for differentiating superior foci from inferior foci. However, several limitations must be considered. Man et al[66] found that the spatial resolution of atrial pace mapping is approximately 17 mm, such that P waves resulting from pacing at sites up to 17 mm apart may be indistinguishable. If the site of atrial tachycardia origin is close to the interatrial septum, the atrium of origin may be easily misclassified. Atrial tachycardias with a right pulmonary vein origin may easily be confused with those of a right atrial origin. However, a monophasic, positive P wave in lead V_1, along with a markedly inferiorly directed P wave axis, is suggestive of a left atrial origin.

Since morphology and polarity of the P wave on the 12-lead ECG are of limited clinical value, the spatial resolution of 62-lead body surface mapping may improve localization of ectopic atrial rhythms. In a recent study, SippensGroenewegen et al[5] performed 62-lead ECG recordings during right atrial pacing at distinct endocardial sites in 9 patients with normal atrial anatomy. P wave integral maps were generated for each paced activation sequence (see Fig. 5B) and were visually selected into 17 groups with nearly identical map features. The spatial resolution of paced P wave body surface mapping in the right atrium was approximately 3.5 cm^2. This database of paced P wave integral maps may provide a clinical tool to perform noninvasive localization of atrial tachycardias before radiofrequency catheter ablation. Another problem that frequently complicates P wave analysis is the superimposition of QRST complexes. A combination of multilead body surface mapping with a QRST subtraction algorithm may facilitate the mapping of the site of origin of even single atrial premature complexes.[7]

Tachycardia-Induced Cardiomyopathy

Heart failure is not infrequently the first manifestation of an incessant atrial tachycardia due to a tachycardia-induced cardiomyopathy, especially in children (Table 3).[60,67-70] Interestingly, patients with continuous atrial tachycardia often present with congestive heart failure and do not have symptomatic palpitations. Presumably, patients with symptomatic atrial tachycardia would be detected earlier, before the onset of congestive heart failure, whereas some "resetting" of the sense of normal

Table 3

Evidence for the Presence of Atrial Tachycardia

Electrocardiographic evidence:
- Repetitive or continuous tachycardia
- Tachycardia with variable R-P interval
- Intermittent AV block ($+/-$ adenosine)

Electrophysiologic evidence:
- Ventricular extrastimulus delivered at the time of His bundle refractoriness does not affect next AA interval
- Ventricular pacing or ventricular extrastimuli results in transient AV block
- Ventricular pacing terminates tachycardia without retrograde atrial activation: exclusion of atrial tachycardia

AV = atrioventricular.

heart beat must be taking place in those presenting with tachymyopathy. Characteristically, the impaired left ventricular function improves and often returns to normal following successful arrhythmia treatment, emphasizing the importance of adequate diagnosis and therapy.[67,69]

Multifocal Atrial Tachycardia

Multifocal atrial tachycardia is considered to be present electrocardiographically if the atrial rate is greater than 100 bpm, and if 3 or more different P wave morphologies may be discerned without a dominant pacemaker, the baseline is isoelectric, and the PP interval is irregularly irregular (Fig. 4).[71] Multifocal atrial tachycardia is found mostly in patients with acute illnesses. The most common

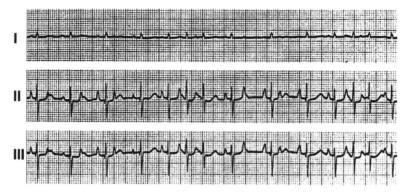

Figure 4. Three surface leads (I, II, and III) in a 68-year-old patient with exacerbation of chronic obstructive lung disease. The P wave rate is faster than 100 bpm (intermittent atrioventricular block), irregularly irregular, and at least 4 different P wave morphologies may be discerned.

cause is chronic obstructive pulmonary disease with or without an acute exacerbation or pneumonia, especially in patients with cor pulmonale.[71] Furthermore, it may be observed after general surgery and a complicated course in the intensive care unit, following exacerbation of congestive heart failure,[72] nonpulmonary infections, diabetes mellitus, coronary artery disease, lung carcinoma, and pulmonary embolus.[73,74] The occurrence of a multifocal atrial tachycardia is frequently associated with hypoxemia and β-adrenergic stimulation, sometimes with hypokalemia and digoxin therapy. As these factors are known to facilitate delayed afterdepolarizations in diseased cardiac muscle, triggered automaticity may be postulated as the underlying mechanism. Finally, in an in vitro study on the effects of theophylline in human atrial tissue, it was found that theophylline may cause delayed afterdepolarizations and triggered arrhythmias.[75] The atrial rate during multifocal atrial tachycardia is usually less than 150 bpm and, therefore, most P waves are conducted through the AV node. Multifocal atrial tachycardia can usually be distinguished from atrial fibrillation by visible P waves, and from sinus tachycardia with frequent premature beats by the absence of a dominant sinus pacemaker. Multifocal atrial tachycardia is associated with a high mortality rate due to the concomitant acute noncardiac conditions, and it almost always resolves with effective treatment of the underlying disease. Symptomatic treatment consists of adequate oxygenation, lowering of sympathomimetic drugs, and correction of metabolic abnormalities. Furthermore, in patients treated with theophylline for their chronic obstructive pulmonary disease and presenting with multifocal atrial tachycardia, theophylline discontinuation has been found to be successful.[76] On rechallenge with increasing doses of theophylline, an increase in ectopic beats was noted until multifocal atrial tachycardia resumed, providing the best evidence of the relationship between theophylline and multifocal atrial tachycardia. As specific antiarrhythmic agents, verapamil, magnesium and also the cardioselective β-blocker metoprolol, if tolerated, have been reported to be effective.[77]

2. Electrophysiologic Characteristics and Diagnosis

Atrial tachycardia is the likely diagnosis if a variable RP tachycardia is present with intermittent AV block, with or without administration of adenosine (see Figs. 6, 9, and 11). However, the RP interval during atrial tachycardia is dependent on the tachycardia rate and AV conduction properties, and AV block may not be observed, as adenosine may cause tachycardia termination before blocking the AV node.

In the electrophysiology laboratory, multisite endocardial pacing and mapping are performed using multiple steerable pacing and recording catheters (see Figs. 17, 23, and 30). Generally, one catheter is positioned in the right ventricular apex in order to perform programmed ventricular stimulation and assess retrograde ventriculoatrial conduction. One multipolar catheter is positioned in the anteroseptal region, where a His recording can be performed (see Figs. 17 and 30). Right atrial pacing can be performed from either a roving catheter positioned in the high right atrium, or a multipolar catheter positioned along the lateral right atrial free wall, on or parallel to the crista terminalis (see Figs. 23 and 30). In this way, the right atrial activation sequence during tachycardia (high right atrium–low right atrium, as during sinus rhythm, or low–high) may be discerned. As a surrogate for the left atrial activation, a multipolar catheter is usually inserted into the coronary sinus (see Figs. 17 and 23). An esophageal electrode may also be useful for recording from the posterior left atrium.

In the electrophysiology laboratory, the diagnosis of atrial tachycardia is based on the exclusion of other tachycardia mechanisms. If there are more atrial activations than ventricular activations, the diagnosis of atrial tachycardia is reasonably assured. If there is an identical number of atrial and ventricular activations, other criteria and maneuvers must be employed. For a long RP tachycardia, the main differential diagnosis is either an atypical (fast–slow or slow–slow) AV nodal reentrant tachycardia or the permanent form of junctional reentrant tachycardia involving a slowly conducting retrograde accessory pathway. For a short RP tachycardia, an accessory pathway and typical AV nodal reentrant tachycardia must be excluded. In order to exclude an accessory pathway, the atrial activation must be dissociated from the ventricular activation. Therefore, the first maneuver consists of introducing progressively earlier premature ventricular beats during tachycardia (Fig. 5A). If one or more premature ventricular beat advances the next atrial activation when the His bundle has been activated, an accessory pathway is present. Sometimes, atrial extrastimuli, double ventricular extrastimuli, or ventricular overdrive pacing must be performed in addition to single ventricular extrastimuli in order to differentiate atrial tachycardia from AV nodal reentry. As shown in Figure 5B, ventricular overdrive pacing was able to dissociate the atrial from the ventricular activation and resulted in AV block. If ventricular overdrive pacing is able to reset the tachycardia, and if the tachycardia resumes after termination of ventricular pacing, an equal number of atrial and ventricular activations is in favor of either AV reentrant tachycardia using an accessory pathway, or AV nodal reentrant tachycardia. If more atrial than ventricular activations are observed, atrial tachycardia is the most likely mechanism, with the rare exception of "double fire" during AV nodal reentrant tachycardia, in which one ventricular beat gives rise to two atrial beats because of successive retrograde conduction over the fast and then the slow pathway. Finally, the mode of tachycardia termination, either spontaneous or following pacing or administration of adenosine, may be helpful. If the tachycardia terminates with the last beat being an atrial activation without ventricular activation, an atrial tachycardia is unlikely. Occasionally, adenosine may affect the AV node at the same time that it affects the

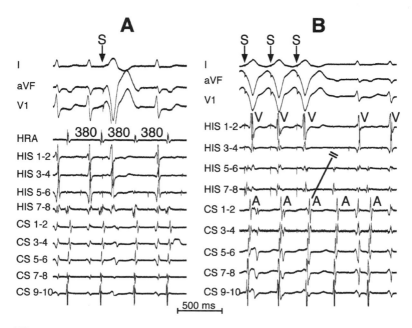

Figure 5. Simultaneous surface ECG (lead I, aVF, V_1) and multisite endocardial recordings during an electrophysiologic study with the attempt to differentiate between atrial tachycardia and atrioventricular nodal reentrant tachycardia. Bipolar endocardial recording is performed from a quadripolar catheter in the high right atrium (HRA), an octopolar catheter in HIS-position (HIS 1–2 = distal/ventricular, His 7–8 = proximal/atrial), and along a decapolar catheter in the coronary sinus (CS; CS 1–2 = distal CS; CS 9–10 = CS os). A. A single early ventricular extrastimulus (S, arrow) does not advance the next atrial activation (HRA) during a supraventricular tachycardia with a cycle length of 380 milliseconds, so the distinction cannot be made. B. Ventricular overdrive pacing (S; arrows), however, resulted in intermittent dissociation of the ventricular (V) activation and the atrial activation (A) with one atrial beat blocked in the AV node, consistent with atrial tachycardia.

tachycardia focus. However, if with repeated injections of adenosine during several episodes of tachycardia the termination is always an atrial activation without a ventricular activation, then atrial tachycardia is very unlikely and AV nodal reentrant tachycardia or an accessory pathway mediated tachycardia is most likely. Whenever ventricular pacing terminates a tachycardia without retrograde activation of the atrium, an atrial tachycardia is excluded and AV nodal reentry or an orthodromic reentrant tachycardia is present.

3. Therapy

Pharmacological treatment of patients with atrial tachycardias has been somewhat disappointing, and there are no controlled trials of medical therapy for atrial tachycardia. Digoxin is frequently used, but it predominantly controls the ventricular response and does not affect the atrial tachycardia itself.[9,60] This is especially true if macroreentry is the underlying mechanism. β-Blockers may be effective in suppressing both paroxysmal and incessant atrial tachycardias due to enhanced automaticity, which are usually catecholamine-sensitive,[78,79] but the overall success rates are low. If triggered automaticity is suggested to be the underlying mechanism, β-blockers and calcium channel blockers should be effective.[35,36] Class Ic antiarrhythmic drugs such as flecainide, encainide, and propafenone have been found to be partially effective for the treatment of atrial tachycardia,[80,81] with efficacy rates of approximately 50%.[82-84] If reentry is the underlying mechanism, Class III antiarrhythmic agents such as amiodarone or sotalol may be superior to Class I drugs, although they are sometimes poorly tolerated or ineffective.[85] Amiodarone has been reported to be effective in both reentrant and automatic atrial tachycardias.[82,86] Atrial tachycardia caused by digitalis intoxication is treated by discontinuation of digitalis, correction of electrolyte and other metabolic disorders, and administration of antidigoxin antibodies. Administration of intravenous potassium, β-blockers, and antiarrhythmic agents such as procainamide have been found to be effective as well.[87,88]

The limited success of pharmacological treatment has prompted the search for a definite cure of this arrhythmia. Several reports describe a high success rate of cardiac surgery with excision of the ectopic focus, especially in children.[60,89] In recent years, with radiofrequency catheter ablation having become standard treatment for AV nodal reentrant tachycardia and Wolff-Parkinson-White (WPW) syndrome, catheter ablation for atrial tachycardia has emerged as a very viable treatment. Table 4 summarizes the results of radiofrequency catheter ablation in patients with atrial tachycardia.[35,50–60] The success rates of radiofrequency catheter ablation vary between 77% and 100%, comparable to results in patients with AV nodal reentrant tachycardia or the WPW syndrome. Therefore, several cases are presented in the following description, with the focus on radiofrequency catheter ablation.

Patient 1, a 43-year-old man without underlying structural heart disease, has had symptomatic palpitations for 6 months, with a significant symptomatic improvement following β-blocker therapy. In the 12-lead ECG (Fig. 6), the presence of a long RP tachycardia (RP interval longer than PR interval) with a rate of 110 bpm suggested an atrial tachycardia as the underlying arrhythmia. The P wave morphology (negative in II, III, and aVF; isoelectric in I, and V_1; and positive in aVR and aVL) suggested a posterior or inferior origin. Subsequently, 62-lead

Table 4

Radiofrequency Catheter Ablation for Atrial Tachycardia

Author (Reference)	Year	Patient Number	Patient Age	Heart Disease # (%)	Tachymy-opathy # (%)	Success # (%)	# Sites	# Right Atrium	# Left Atrium
Kalman (50)	1998	27	41 ± 14	1 (4)	2 (8)	29/31 (94)	31	27	4
Pappone (51)	1996	45	29 ± 11	23 (51)	—	42/45 (93)	45	36	9
Poty (52)	1996	36	40 ± 18	13 (36)	—	31/36 (86)	36	33	3
Tang (53)	1995	31	39 ± 20	9 (29)	4 (13)	31/31 (100)	31	17	14
Feld (54)	1995	10	51 ± 17	5 (50)	—	10/10 (100)	10	9	1
Chen (35)	1994	36	57 ± 13	9 (25)	—	32/34 (94)	43	36	7
Lesh (55)	1994	11	31 ± 23	2 (18)	5 (45)	11/12 (92)	12	7	5
Goldberger (56)	1993	13	38 ± 22	3 (23)	4 (31)	10/13 (77)	13	13	0
Kay (57)	1993	11	43 ± 30	2 (18)	2 (18)	10/11 (91)	11	9	2
Tracy (58)	1993	10	32 ± 11	2 (20)	—	9/11 (81)	11	9	2
Walsh (59)	1992	12	12 ± 5	0	12 (100)	11/12 (82)	12	5	7
Gillette (60)	1985	16	10 ± 4	0	10 (63)	13/16 (81)	16	10	6

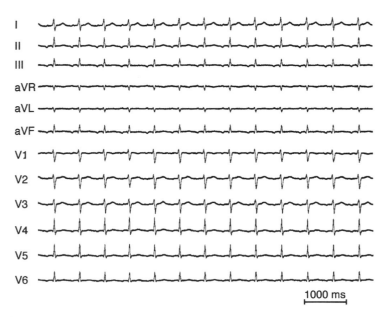

Figure 6. Twelve-lead ECG during supraventricular tachycardia in patient 1, demonstrating a long RP tachycardia with positive P waves in I, aVR, and aVL, negative P waves in II, III, and aVF, and biphasic in lead V_1.

body surface mapping was performed. Figure 7 demonstrates the lead distribution and the P wave integral map during tachycardia. After comparison of the P wave integral map with a right atrial database,[5] the most probable location was suggested to be in the low posteroseptal right atrium. Note that the P wave minimum is located on the

$\longrightarrow$

Figure 7. Diagram of the 62 lead sites superimposed over the human torso (A) and the P wave integral map during atrial tachycardia (B) in patient 1. The electrode array contains the standard 6 precordial leads (open circles overlying the heart). The V_4 lead tracing below the map demonstrates the interval over which the integral was *(continued)*

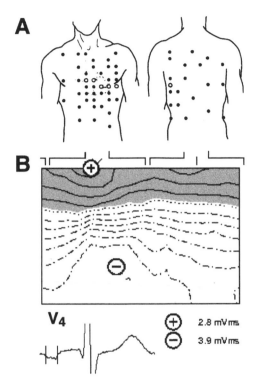

Figure 7. *continued*   computed (area between two vertical bars) during tachycardia. The map is represented as an unrolled cylinder opened at the level of the right posterior axilla with the left and right sides of the map corresponding to the front and back of the chest, respectively. The locations of the sternum (left) and spine (right) are marked schematically above the map. Positive (gray area) and negative (white area) isointegral lines are indicated by solid and dashed lines, respectively; the zero line is marked by the dotted line. The increment between the isointegral lines is linear and varies in accordance to the absolute positive or negative voltage amplitudes. Plus and minus signs depict the location of the maximum and minimum, respectively; their amplitudes are given below the map. The electromotive forces during this ectopic atrial excitation sequence are oriented in a superior and slightly rightward direction. By comparing the patient's P wave integral map with the right atrial database,[5] the origin of the atrial tachycardia was in the low posteroseptal right atrium, close to the os of the coronary sinus.

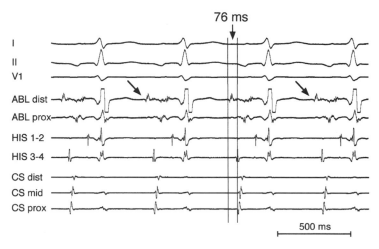

Figure 8. Surface ECG and endocardial recordings during electrophysiologic study and mapping of atrial tachycardia in patient 1. On the tip of the ablation catheter (ABL dist; site of successful ablation), a low-amplitude, fragmented signal can be observed (arrow). The onset of the fragmented signal is 76 milliseconds earlier than the onset of the surface P wave in lead II and significantly earlier than any other endocardial activation, either along the interatrial septum (HIS) or along the coronary sinus (CS; dist = distal CS; prox = proximal CS, CS os). Application of radiofrequency energy to this site resulted in termination of atrial tachycardia, which could no longer be induced.

lower portion of the chest, just left of midline, with the P wave integral vector (from minimum to maximum) pointing toward the right shoulder. Subsequent right atrial endocardial mapping revealed the earliest activation during atrial tachycardia in the low posteroseptal right atrium. Figure 8 demonstrates a low-amplitude, fragmented signal on the distal tip of the ablation catheter, 76 milliseconds earlier than the P wave onset in lead II, and considerably earlier than any other endocardial recording (atrial signal on the HIS and proximal coronary sinus catheter). During the first radiofrequency application, the tachycardia terminated and was no longer inducible, despite an aggressive stimulation protocol and administration of catecholamines.

Patient 2 is a 29-year-old woman without structural heart disease and with a 2-year history of palpitations. In a prior electrophysiologic study, dual AV node physiology and a concealed bypass tract had been excluded, and no sustained arrhythmia was inducible. As the patient remained highly symptomatic, she was scheduled for a restudy, and on the day of hospital admission, she was found to be in a sustained supraventricular tachycardia. The 12-lead ECG (Fig. 9) demonstrates regular P waves at a rate

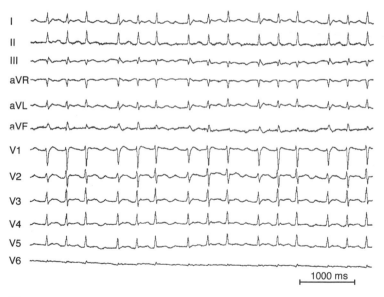

Figure 9. Twelve-lead ECG during supraventricular tachycardia in patient 2, with regular P waves at a rate of approximately 200 bpm, positive in I, aVL, and V_1 through V_4, negative in III, aVR, and aVF, and a 4:3 atrioventricular conduction.

of approximately 200 bpm and a 4:3 AV conduction. The fact that the ventricle was not required for tachycardia sustenance is suggestive of an atrial tachycardia as the underlying mechanism. The P wave morphology was not diagnostic of either a right or left atrial focus. As no sufficiently early activation was found during right atrial mapping, a transseptal procedure was performed. The earliest activation during atrial tachycardia was found in the left upper pulmonary vein, 55 milliseconds before the onset of the surface P wave (Fig. 10). The tachycardia terminated

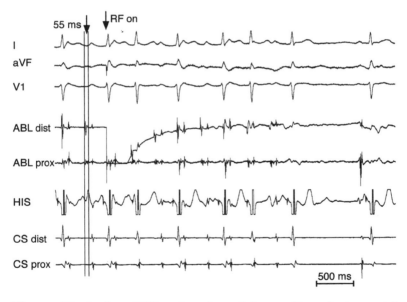

Figure 10. Surface ECG and endocardial recordings during atrial tachycardia and radiofrequency application (RF on; arrow) in patient 2. On the tip of the ablation catheter, a distinct signal 55 milliseconds earlier than the onset of the surface P wave can be observed. Termination of atrial tachycardia 2.5 seconds after initiation of radiofrequency application, followed by sinus rhythm.

2.5 seconds after the initiation of radiofrequency application and was no longer inducible despite an aggressive stimulation protocol and infusion of isoproterenol.

Patient 3 is a 72-year-old female with a history of increasingly frequent episodes of palpitations. The patient was admitted with continuous supraventricular tachycardia. The 12-lead ECG (Fig. 11) demonstrates again a long RP tachycardia, and the occurrence of high-grade AV block without tachycardia termination following intravenous administration of adenosine proves the presence of an atrial tachycardia. The P wave morphology, which could be clearly appreciated after adenosine administration (negative in II, III, aVF, and V_1; isoelectric in I; and positive in aVR and aVL) was consistent with a low right atrial focus. Endocardial mapping revealed the earliest atrial activation during tachycardia on the inferior crista terminalis. The tachycardia terminated within the first 3 seconds of radiofrequency energy application (Fig. 12), and was no longer inducible.

Patient 4 is a 41-year-old female with a long history of palpitations. She was found to have dual AV node physiology and underwent successful slow pathway ablation, but remained symptomatic for palpitations, significantly influencing her activity level. A 24-hour Holter recording was consistent with presumed inappropriate sinus tachycardia based on the P wave morphology similar to sinus rhythm. Therefore, the patient was referred for sinus node modification. A baseline electrophysiologic study was performed, but was unrevealing. Increasing doses of isoproterenol (up to 4 μg/min), combined with atropine 0.5 mg revealed a physiologic increase in the sinus rate (maximum, 160 bpm). However, nonsustained episodes of atrial

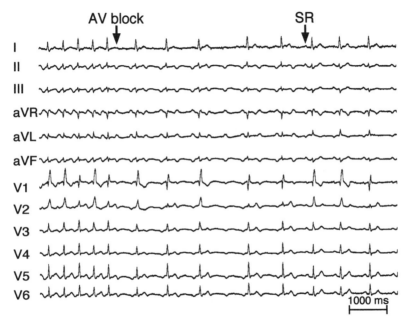

Figure 11. Twelve-lead ECG during supraventricular tachycardia with a rate of 160 bpm in patient 3 during administration of 12 mg of adenosine. First, 1:1 atrioventricular (AV) conduction during tachycardia with a right bundle branch block aberrance is observed. The adenosine effect causes 2:1 and 3:1 AV block (arrow), clearly unmasking negative P waves in II, III, aVF, and V_1, positive P waves in aVR and aVL, and isoelectric in lead I. Subsequently, the tachycardia terminates, and sinus rhythm (SR) with intermittent right bundle branch block aberrance is present.

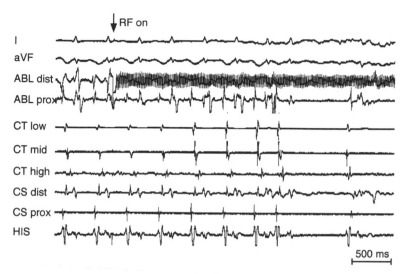

Figure 12. Surface ECG and endocardial recordings during atrial tachycardia and radiofrequency application (RF on; arrow) in patient 3. The earliest activation during atrial tachycardia was found to be on the low crista terminalis (CT). Atrial tachycardia terminated 3.0 seconds after initiation of radiofrequency application with an atrial premature beat and could no longer be induced. CT = bipolar recordings on a 20-pole catheter along the crista terminalis (low, mid, and high).

tachycardia were reproducibly inducible with atrial overdrive pacing (Fig. 13A). Right atrial mapping was performed, and the earliest activation was found to be in the area of the high crista terminalis (Fig. 13B). Intracardiac echocardiography was performed to visualize this region (Fig. 14). Good wall contact was confirmed with intracardiac ultrasound, and several radiofrequency applications were performed during sinus rhythm. Subsequently, no further episodes of atrial tachycardia were induced de-

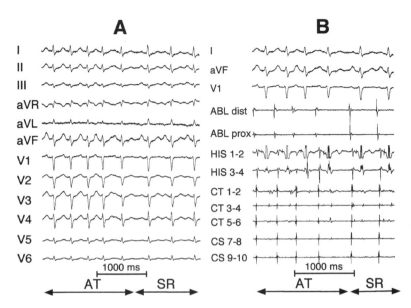

Figure 13. Twelve-lead surface ECG (A) and surface ECG and endocardial recordings (B) during the termination of an episode of atrial tachycardia in patient 4. Earliest activation during atrial tachycardia was found to be in the area of the high crista terminalis (B, left), very similar to the activation sequence during sinus rhythm (B, right), although careful measurement reveals that the roving ablation catheter records an activation time relation to other atrial sites which is slightly earlier during the atrial tachycardia than it is during sinus rhythm.

spite atrial pacing and increasing doses of isoproterenol. Furthermore, the maximum heart rate on 4 μg of isoproterenol was lowered to 135 bpm.

One limitation of ablation of focal atrial tachycardia in the electrophysiology laboratory is that the tachycardia may not be constantly present or easily provoked with catecholamines or pacing. Thus, the electrophysiol-

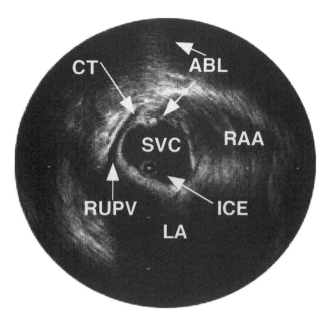

Figure 14. Intracardiac echocardiography image of the high right atrium. The image shows the echocardiography probe (ICE) in the superior vena cava (SVC) right at the junction to the right atrium, with the right atrial appendage (RAA) to the right. The tip of the ablation catheter (ABL) with the characteristic fan-shaped artifact (arrows) is in contact with the high crista terminalis (CT). LA = left atrium; RUPV = right upper pulmonary vein.

ogist may have only brief bursts of atrial tachycardia to map. One tool that can be of assistance in this setting is electroanatomic mapping using a nonfluoroscopic system. This allows a composite activation map to be developed over time, and ablation to be performed at the site of earliest activation. Such was the case in patient 5, a 47-year-old female with persistent palpitations due to

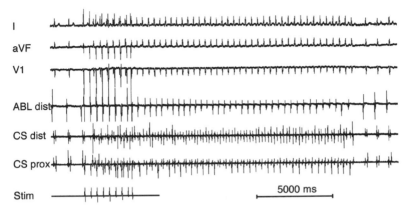

I

aVF

V1

ABL dist

CS dist

CS prox

Stim   5000 ms

Figure 15. Surface ECG and endocardial recording during a brief paroxysm of atrial tachycardia, induced with programmed electrical stimulation, as shown on the stimulation (Stim) channel.

intermittent atrial tachycardia following a successful prior atrial flutter ablation. Figure 15 shows a rare episode of nonsustained atrial tachycardia inducible with programmed stimulation. Conventional mapping of the right atrium suggested a mid right atrial focus of atrial tachycardia, but confirmation of this, sufficient to target radiofrequency energy application, was not possible due to the rare tachycardia episodes and the subsequent lack of catheter stability during continuous attempts to induce tachycardia. Figure 16 shows the nonfluoroscopic electroanatomic map. The red color demonstrates early activation in the area of the mid crista terminalis. Several radiofrequency applications were performed in the area of the mid crista terminalis and, subsequently, no further tachycardia was inducible or occurred spontaneously.

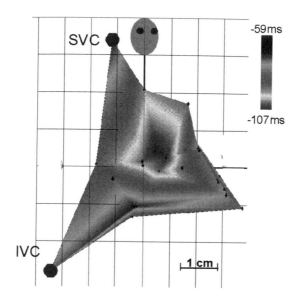

Figure 16. Right anterior oblique view of the nonfluoroscopic, electroanatomic map of the right atrium during nonsustained atrial tachycardia, using the CARTO system, in patient 5. The earliest activation during atrial tachycardia (red; − 59 milliseconds, as compared to the reference signal, a bipolar recording in the proximal coronary sinus) is found on the mid anterolateral right atrium. The subsequent endocardial activation progresses radially from this focus. Ablation at this site of early activation, guided by electroanatomic mapping, was successful in preventing further paroxysms of atrial tachycardia. See color plate.

The Role of Newer Technologies for Mapping and Ablation of Atrial Tachycardia

Use of fluoroscopy for catheter localization is satisfactory for most standard ablative procedures. However, endocardial anatomic structures such as the crista terminalis or the pulmonary vein ostia play an important role in atrial tachycardias and are not distinguishable with fluoroscopy alone. In addition, fluoroscopy exposure times often exceed 1 hour, even for standard ablative procedures. Therefore, intracardiac echocardiography has been used to provide direct endocardial visualization during electrophysiologic study and ablation, especially in patients with atrial tachycardia.[2–4,50]

Current and future potential uses of intracardiac ultrasound imaging for electrophysiologic evaluation and therapy of atrial tachycardias are summarized in Table 5. Intracardiac echocardiography allows for precise localization of the ablation catheter tip in relation to endocardial structures such as crista terminalis, eustachian ridge, fossa ovalis, and coronary sinus os (see Figs. 14 and 30). There is increasing evidence to suggest that the substrate for a variety of arrhythmias, especially atrial tachycardia and focal atrial fibrillation, may be anatomically determined, possibly allowing for guidance of the ablative procedure by anatomic landmarks. For right atrial tachycardias, the crista terminalis has been found to be a

Table 5

Use of Intracardiac Echocardiography for Evaluation and Therapy of Atrial Tachycardia

1) Localization of the catheter tip in relation to endocardial structures
2) Reduction of fluoroscopy time
3) Evaluation of catheter tip-tissue contact
4) Confirmation and identification of lesion size
5) Early identification of complications
6) Assistance in guidance of transseptal puncture
7) Repositioning of catheter to same site after dislodgement

preferential site of origin.[50] The sinus node pacemaker complex has been found to be distributed over a wide area along the crista terminalis.[30,31] Successful modification of the sinus node for treatment of inappropriate sinus tachycardia may be achieved by creating a set of lesions, targeted along the crista terminalis from high anteromedial and progressing inferiorly, guided by intracardiac echocardiography. Before radiofrequency application, tissue contact can be assessed, and following radiofrequency application, lesion size and continuity can be identified.[4] On occasion, intracardiac ultrasound may provide early detection of complications; clot formation can be detected and early pericardial tamponade can be visualized. Transseptal puncture may be difficult to perform in patients with distorted anatomy, and intracardiac ultrasound may provide direct visualization of the fossa ovalis and the needle tenting the fossa. Furthermore, new technology, especially phased-array imaging, may facilitate visualization of left atrial structures from the right atrium. Visualization of left atrial structures such as the pulmonary veins may possibly further improve our understanding of the role of endocardial structures in atrial arrhythmogenesis. Finally, improved technology may facilitate creation of continuous transmural long linear lesions in both right and left atrium for a catheter-based cure for atrial fibrillation.[90,91]

Current single-beat, multielectrode mapping techniques during atrial tachycardia may be difficult and time consuming. Recent studies[92-94] suggest that a basket catheter with multiple splines and electrodes may facilitate mapping of right atrial tachycardias. Figure 17 shows the fluoroscopic image of a basket catheter with 8 splines and 8 electrodes on each spline. In this fashion, multipolar 3-dimensional recording of right atrial tachycardias has

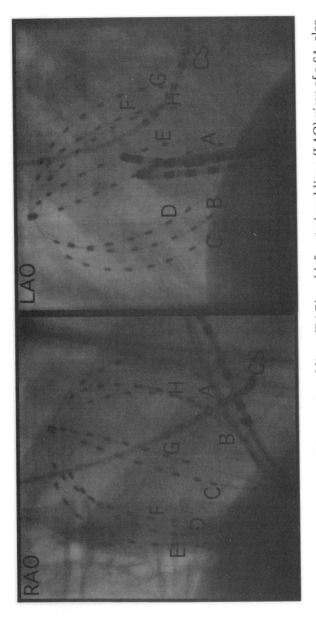

Figure 17. Fluoroscopic right anterior oblique (RAO) and left anterior oblique (LAO) view of a 64–electrode basket catheter (Constellation, EPT, Boston Scientific, Watertown, MA) inserted into the right atrium. Individual splines are labeled with letters from A to H. On each spline, 8 electrodes are represented as radiopaque markers. Furthermore, a multipolar catheter is inserted into the coronary sinus (CS), one catheter is positioned along the anteroseptal right atrium in HIS position, and one catheter is inserted into the right ventricular apex. Figure shown, with permission, from References 92 through 94.

been facilitated in the clinical electrophysiology laboratory. Although the analysis of 64 channels may be challenging, automated analysis with computer-assisted animation may improve localization and reduce mapping time of focal atrial arrhythmias.

A method for electroanatomic catheter-based mapping of the heart (CARTO system, Biosense Inc., Tel Aviv, Israel) was recently introduced, which may overcome some of the shortcomings of traditional mapping.[95–97] A high-resolution miniature location sensor is mounted at the tip of a standard, deflectable ablation catheter. The location and orientation of the sensor is determined by integrating the sensed electromagnetic fields to a set of known radiated fields. The system reconstructs a 3-dimensional map from endocardial sites that have been sequentially mapped. Furthermore, individual local activation times are determined for every mapped site with respect to a predetermined reference time. The local activation times are provided in a variety of formats, such as a color-coded isochronal map, and the electrophysiologic information is superimposed on the anatomy of the respective mapped areas of the heart chamber.

Recent studies[98–100] have demonstrated spatial and temporal accuracy and reproducibility and initial clinical utility. The reliable renavigation of the ablation catheter to a site that had been identified earlier seems to be of advantage in selected cases. After the collection of a number of mapping points, the focus can be identified during mapping of even brief episodes of atrial tachycardia, as the site with the earliest local activation time, relative to a predetermined reference time. Subsequently, accurate renavigation, according to the 3-dimensional map of the chamber, can be attempted during sinus rhythm, followed by radiofrequency application. This nonfluoroscopic electroanatomic mapping system may also potentially be of benefit for patients with atrial arrhythmias and complex anatomy, such as incisional intraatrial reentrant tachycardias following corrective surgery of congenital heart disease (see Section VI and Figs. 26 and 27).[37,101] Surgical conduction barriers such as conduits and patches can be identified as electrically silent areas (very low voltage, farfield signals) using a color-coded "voltage map," and surgical incisions can be identified as double potentials (see Figs. 26 and 27). Subsequent activation mapping allows demonstration of the reentrant circuit and a protected isthmus.

While electroanatomic mapping offers an advantage in patients with nonsustained arrhythmias, mapping still requires contact of the catheter with the earliest site of endocardial activation. Greater speed might be achieved and the ability to map brief tachycardias enhanced with a multipoint noncontact electrode.[102-104] In recent reports of such a noncontact mapping system,[102-104] a catheter-mounted noncontact multielectrode array was inserted in the left ventricle or right atrium in patients with a variety of arrhythmias. The mapping catheter was a 64-wire braid around an 8-mL balloon on a 9F catheter. Subsequently, mathematical reconstruction of more than 3300 electrograms was performed, and the electrograms were superimposed onto a computer model of the endocardium, creating isopotential and isochronal maps. In patients with ventricular tachycardia,[103] the exit site was identified in a high percentage, facilitating radiofrequency ablation. In patients with atrial flutter,[102] the flutter circuit and the specific effect of previous failed radiofrequency catheter ablation were demonstrated. Further prospective studies in more patients will determine ultimate clinical utility of this promising tool.

The Role of Atrial Anatomy

It is remarkable that the sites of tachycardia origin and subsequent successful radiofrequency catheter ablation are not randomly distributed over both right and left atrium.[35,50-60] Certain anatomic structures, such as the crista terminalis, orifice of right or left atrial appendage, coronary sinus os, and the pulmonary veins in the left atrium, are frequently reported as tachycardia origins. In Figure 18, tachycardia foci are represented in the schematic drawing of the right and left atrium, based on several clinical reports (Table 4). Note that 85% of the left atrial tachycardias are located at 5 distinct sites, and that 38% of the specified right atrial tachycardia sites could be assigned to 3 distinct right atrial sites. Recently, Kalman et al[50] showed that the crista terminalis is a frequent site of origin for right atrial tachycardias.

The anatomic preference may be due to the necessity of both cells with abnormal automaticity, and a region of poor cell-to-cell coupling, in order to manifest abnormal firing.[39,49] For example, the orifices of vessels such as the pulmonary veins or the superior vena cava may represent border zones, with the bulk of atrial muscle suddenly decreasing and thinning as they spread along the vessel wall. Regardless of the exact underlying mechanism, however, the knowledge about anatomic preferences may help to guide radiofrequency catheter ablation, especially if induction or maintenance of tachycardia in the electrophysiology laboratory is difficult.

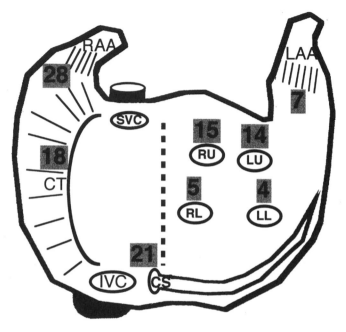

RA, other sites: n=108   LA, other sites: n=8

Figure 18. Schematic of the right atrium (RA) and the left atrium (LA), with preferential sites of origin of focal atrial tachycardias from a compendium of clinical reports. Preferential sites were found to be the orifice of the right atrial appendage (RAA, n = 28), along the crista terminalis (CT; n = 18, although the crista terminalis was not identified in most studies), and the os of the coronary sinus (CS; n = 21) in the right atrium. In the left atrium, preferential sites were found to be the right upper pulmonary vein (RU; n = 15), the left upper pulmonary vein (LU; n = 14), the right lower pulmonary vein (RL; n = 5), the left lower pulmonary vein (LL; n = 4) and the orifice of the left atrial appendage (LAA; n = 7). IVC = inferior vena cava; SVC = superior vena cava.

V. Atrial Fibrillation as a Manifestation of Focal Atrial Activation

Atrial fibrillation has long been considered to be maintained by multiple reentrant wavelets.[105] After the high success rate of a surgical procedure to cure atrial fibrillation,[106,107] attempts have been made to cure atrial fibrillation with radiofrequency catheter ablation, based on the surgical "Maze procedure." While these early studies suffered from low success rates and high complication rates,[108,109] it has been observed that in patients with paroxysmal atrial fibrillation, an underlying focus of a rapid atrial tachycardia was frequently unmasked after linear lesion creation.[109] Furthermore, if the rapidly firing focus, frequently located within one of the pulmonary veins, could be abolished with focal application of radiofrequency energy, the result was no further episodes of atrial fibrillation.[110] These initial findings have been extended to a larger number of patients, thus providing an etiologic link between atrial tachycardia and the most common atrial arrhythmia, atrial fibrillation. This is particularly exciting, since it implies that atrial fibrillation can be cured with focal radiofrequency application.[111]

The relevance of a rapidly firing focus in the general population of patients with atrial fibrillation is still unknown. Likewise, even in patients with focally triggered atrial fibrillation, the mechanism of atrial fibrillation maintenance has yet to be determined. On the one hand, the focal trigger may only be essential for initiation of atrial fibrillation, and atrial fibrillation is subsequently maintained by multiple reentrant wavelets facilitated by short- and long-term electrical remodeling.[112,113] On the other hand, it may be hypothesized that at least in some patients with structurally normal hearts and paroxysmal atrial fibrillation, atrial fibrillation may not only be "focally triggered," but also "focally driven." In other words, the rapid focal activity is essential for initiation *and* maintenance of atrial fibrillation.

1. Clinical and Electrocardiographic Presentation

To date, those patients with paroxysmal atrial fibrillation who have had a documented underlying focal atrial trigger have usually had frequent (more than once a week) episodes of atrial fibrillation as well as frequent atrial ectopic beats, documented on a 24-hour Holter recording. If it is possible to discern the P wave morphology, isolated ectopic atrial beats as well as the premature beats triggering atrial fibrillation have a very similar P wave morphology.

2. Electrophysiologic Characteristics and Diagnosis

The patient history, the 12-lead ECG, and the finding of multiple paroxysms of atrial fibrillation and frequent atrial premature beats during Holter monitoring are very suggestive of a "focal" trigger for atrial fibrillation. The electrophysiologic study and subsequent catheter mapping can confirm the presence of a single, rapidly firing focus triggering atrial fibrillation; in some cases there may be more than one focus. As recent data have elegantly shown, 94% of the focal triggers arose from the pulmonary veins—sometimes up to 4 cm away from the junction of the pulmonary vein and left atrium. There are, however, several important limitations to our present approach to radiofrequency catheter ablation of focal atrial fibrillation (Table 6): 1) It can be very difficult to induce focal sources in the electrophysiology laboratory. In most cases, these focal sources do not respond to pacing maneuvers or chemical alterations in autonomic tone, such as administration of catecholamines. Therefore, the frustrating situation is all too common: despite a characteristic clinical profile and documented frequent monomorphic atrial premature beats triggering atrial fibrillation, the patient does not demonstrate adequate spontaneous arrhythmia for mapping during the electrophysiologic study. 2) Pulmonary veins have a complex, 3-dimensional branching structure, and the focus triggering onset of atrial fibrillation is usually found 2 to 4 cm inside one of the pulmonary veins.[114] Thus, detailed mapping is frequently difficult, even if the focal trigger is constantly firing, which is generally not the case. 3) Ongoing atrial fibrillation masks any focal trigger and makes it difficult to map the trigger.[110,111] Multiple external or internal defibrillations, sometimes combined with antiarrhythmic drugs, may be necessary

Table 6

Limitations of Mapping and Ablation of Focal Atrial Fibrillation Using Standard Techniques

---

1) No reproducible method of induction of focal triggers
2) Unpredictability of spontaneous firing
3) Three-dimensional branching structure of pulmonary veins
4) Sustained atrial fibrillation masks focal trigger
5) Endpoint of ablation is difficult to assess
6) Multiple pulmonary vein foci

---

in order to perform adequate mapping. 4) Due to the spontaneous variability of firing of the focus, the endpoint in the electrophysiology laboratory is difficult to define. 5) In approximately 30% of patients, more than one pulmonary vein focus is present. Therefore, even if history and ambulatory monitoring results are promising and justify an attempt of radiofrequency catheter ablation for a focally triggered atrial fibrillation, the physician and patient must be aware of present limitations. Novel technology such as anatomically based electrical isolation of a pulmonary vein from the left atrium may be promising,[115] but further studies must address efficacy and safety and, in particular, the occurrence of pulmonary stenosis.

3. Therapy

Examples of successfully treated patients are shown in Figures 19 through 22. Patient 6 is a 40-year-old male without underlying structural heart disease and with a history of frequent episodes of palpitations associated with lightheadedness. A 24-hour Holter monitor showed frequent premature atrial beats (more than 4000/24 hours) as well as nonsustained episodes of atrial fibrillation. Figure 19 shows onset and termination of an episode of nonsustained atrial fibrillation during Holter monitoring. In addition to two surface leads, we have included an esophageal probe, which allows recording from the posterior left atrium, very near the pulmonary veins. Of note is that the earliest activation of the atrial premature beat triggering atrial fibrillation is on the esophageal lead, significantly earlier than the surface P wave, suggesting a left posterior atrial origin consistent with a trigger in the

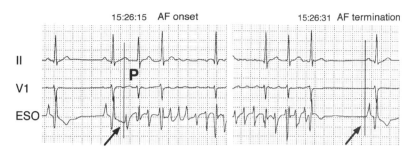

Figure 19. Onset (left panel, 15:26:15) and termination (right panel, 15:26:31) of an episode of nonsustained atrial fibrillation (AF) in patient 1 during 24-hour Holter recording. Shown are surface leads II and V_1, and a third electrode that has been modified as a bipolar esophageal recording (ESO). The activation on the esophageal electrode during the atrial premature beat triggering onset of atrial fibrillation (arrow, left panel) is found to be considerably earlier than the positive P wave in lead V1 (P, black bar), whereas during sinus rhythm, the P wave in lead II is on time with the esophageal recording (arrow, black bar right panel).

pulmonary vein. Figure 20 shows the 12-lead ECG, demonstrating two nonsustained episodes of atrial fibrillation. Figure 21 shows surface and endocardial recordings during mapping of focally triggered atrial fibrillation. One sinus beat is followed by a burst of focal firing. The ablation catheter is positioned in the left upper pulmonary vein. It is of note that during the first sinus beat, a sharp potential on the ablation catheter (arrow) follows the initial, low-amplitude signal. During the premature atrial beats, however, the sharp potential is significantly earlier than any other endocardial recording sites, including the posteroseptal right atrium, along the crista terminalis and along the coronary sinus. The esophageal signal is almost on time with the early signal on the ablation catheter. Radiofrequency energy was applied at this spot in the left

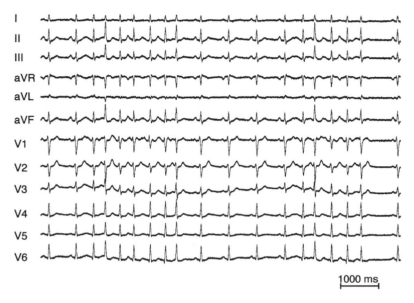

Figure 20. Twelve-lead ECG in patient 6 with paroxysmal atrial fibrillation. Onset and termination of two brief episodes of atrial fibrillation are shown.

upper pulmonary vein, and despite administration of catecholamines, no further ectopy was observed. The patient remains free of atrial fibrillation in follow-up.

Patient 7 is a 49-year-old male with a 6-year history of atrial fibrillation who has failed a total of 4 antiarrhythmic drugs. Prior to the onset of atrial fibrillation, which lasts up to 1 or 2 days, the patient has always noticed skipped heart beats. A Holter recording demonstrated multiple atrial premature beats, which all seemed to have the same morphology. At the beginning of the electrophysiologic study, the patient was found to be in atrial fibrillation. Therefore, an external atrial defibrillation was performed, but atrial fibrillation recurred after several sinus

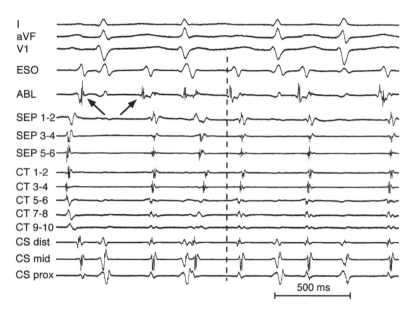

Figure 21. Surface and endocardial recordings during mapping of focal atrial fibrillation in patient 6. During mapping, the tip of the ablation catheter is in the left upper pulmonary vein. Other catheters used for mapping are a multipolar catheter along the posteroseptal right atrium (SEP), a multipolar catheter along the crista terminalis (CT; CT 9–10 = high crista, CT 1–2 = low crista terminalis), and a multipolar coronary sinus catheter (CS; CS prox = close to the CS os). A sharp, fragmented potential is observed on the ablation catheter, late, and at the end of the surface P wave during sinus rhythm (first beat, arrow). However, during the subsequent 4 beats of rapid focal atrial tachycardia, the fragmented signal is found to be significantly earlier than any other endocardial activation (dashed line). Of notice, the second earliest activation is found on the esophageal lead, still significantly earlier than any other endocardial activation on the right side (SEP, CT) or along the coronary sinus (CS).

beats. After two more cardioversions and subsequent early recurrence of atrial fibrillation, 1 mg of ibutilide was administered. Sustained atrial fibrillation terminated, but frequent atrial premature beats and nonsustained episodes of atrial tachycardia and atrial fibrillation still occurred, allowing atrial mapping. Figure 22 shows the en-

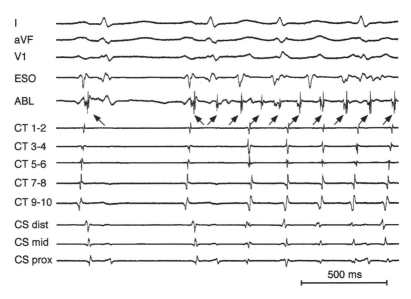

Figure 22. Surface and endocardial recordings during mapping of focal atrial fibrillation in patient 7. During mapping, the tip of the ablation catheter is in the right upper pulmonary vein. Again, a discrete, fragmented potential is observed on the ablation catheter toward the end of the surface P wave during sinus rhythm (first two beats, arrows). This high-frequency spike likely represents late activation in the right upper pulmonary vein. The initial, somewhat farfield deflection represents activation of the surrounding left atrium. During the subsequent beats of rapid focal atrial tachycardia, this discrete, high-frequency signal appears much earlier than any other endocardial activation. Furthermore, variable exit block from the site of origin in the right upper pulmonary vein to the right atrium (crista terminalis, CT) and left atrium (coronary sinus, CS) is noted.

docardial activation sequence during onset of nonsustained atrial fibrillation. The ablation catheter was located in the right upper pulmonary vein. Subsequently, the ablation catheter recorded a rapid focal atrial tachycardia with a cycle length of approximately 160 milliseconds. However, the rest of the atrium could not follow 1:1, and intermittent 2:1 exit block from the rapidly firing focus into the left and right atrium was observed. Mapping during atrial tachycardia as well as atrial premature beats confirmed this site to be earliest. Figure 23 shows the fluoroscopic image of the catheter position. Of note, the tip of the ablation catheter at the site of subsequent successful radiofrequency ablation is well within the right upper pulmonary vein and well outside the cardiac silhouette.

This anatomic predominance of sites of origin of focal triggers of atrial fibrillation is striking (Fig. 24); in the recently reported 45 patients, 65 out of 69 focal triggers (94%) arose from the pulmonary veins, 48 of them from one of the upper pulmonary veins. Sparce, highly anisotropic atrial fibers extending well onto the body of the pulmonary veins have been demonstrated and may be the substrate for the focal trigger.[114,116] A number of factors such as stretch,[117] fibrosis, ischemia, variations in autonomic tone,[118,119] or the changes induced by atrial fibrillation itself[112,113] may further influence the propensity for the focal trigger to fire. The relevance of a focal trigger has been clearly demonstrated for a subset of patients with very frequent paroxysms of atrial fibrillation. It is intriguing to speculate that patients with less frequent paroxysmal atrial fibrillation, or even those with persistent or chronic atrial fibrillation, may have a focal trigger. Further research will be needed in order to determine the true incidence of focal triggers in the larger group of patients

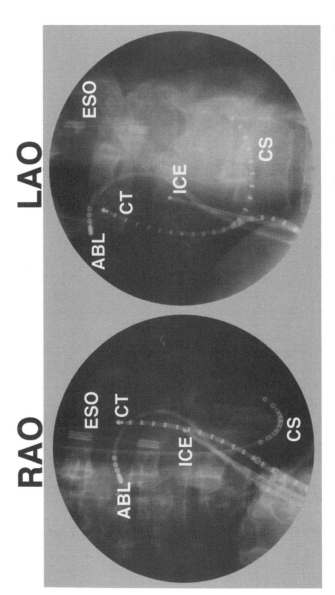

Figure 23. Fluoroscopic right anterior oblique (RAO) and left anterior oblique (LAO) view of the catheter position during mapping of focally triggered atrial fibrillation in patient 7 with a right upper pulmonary vein trigger for atrial fibrillation. The ablation catheter (ABL) is well within the right upper pulmonary vein at least 4 cm from the left atrial-pulmonary vein junction. CS = decapolar catheter in the coronary sinus; CT = 20-pole catheter along the crista terminalis; ESO = bipolar esophageal recording catheter; ICE = tip of the intracardiac echocardiography catheter.

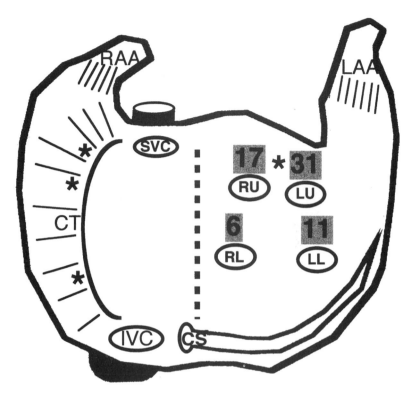

Figure 24. Schematic of the right atrium (RA) and the left atrium (LA), with preferential sites of origin of focal atrial fibrillation triggers according to the reported sites of successful radiofrequency catheter ablation. Except for 5 (7%) foci arising near the crista terminalis (CT; asterisks), focal triggers were found to be the left upper pulmonary vein (LU; n = 31, 45%), the right upper pulmonary vein (RU; n = 17, 25%), the left lower pulmonary vein (LL; n = 11, 16%), and the right lower pulmonary vein (RL; n = 6, 9%). CS = coronary sinus; IVC = inferior vena cava; LAA = left atrial appendage; RAA = right atrial appendage; SVC = superior vena cava.

with persistent or infrequently paroxysmal atrial fibrillation.

VI. Incisional Intraatrial Reentrant Tachycardia

Although reentry may frequently serve as an underlying mechanism for atrial tachycardias without prior cardiac surgery, clinical presentation and subsequent therapy of "incisional" reentrant atrial tachycardia following surgery for congenital heart disease is so specific that it warrants coverage in a separate section. As children undergoing repair or palliation of a congenital heart disease have benefited with an increasing survival rate, the incidence and spectrum of cardiac arrhythmias are gradually changing.[120] Multiple palliative and corrective cardiac surgeries for congenital heart disease result in surgical incisions and other conduction barriers such as conduits and patches for closure of defects.[37,55,121–123] Together with natural anatomic obstacles, such as orifices of great vessels and AV annulus, these conduction barriers may facilitate intraatrial reentry (see Fig. 1). The reentrant activation wavefront during tachycardia may circle around conduction barriers, and in addition, anatomic barriers protect the wavefront from lateral collision that would otherwise terminate reentry.

Following surgery for congenital heart disease, a variety of arrhythmias can complicate the procedure. Early atrial tachyarrhythmias, complete AV block, and junctional ectopic tachycardia are beyond the scope of this volume, as are early and late ventricular tachyarrhythmias. Therefore, the following description focuses on late intraatrial reentrant tachycardias following corrective surgery for congenital heart disease.

1. Clinical and Electrocardiographic Presentation

Incisional intraatrial reentrant tachycardia following repair or palliation of congenital heart disease is a common and potentially serious complication. Table 7 summarizes recent studies[37,55,121-123] of patients with incisional intraatrial reentrant tachycardia, focusing on radiofrequency catheter ablation. The long mean duration of symptoms (0.5 to 8.8 years) and the high mean number of failed antiarrhythmic drugs (2.1 to 3.6) imply that this series represents a quite selected subset of patients. Out of the 58 patients, the underlying surgery or congenital

Table 7

Radiofrequency Catheter Ablation for Incisional Reentrant
Atrial Tachycardia

Author (Reference)	Year	Patient Number	Patient Age (y)	Symptom Duration (y)	Drugs Failed (#)	Acute Success # (%)
Kalman et al (37)	1996	18	27 ± 15	7.3 ± 5.2	3.5 ± 1.4	15/18 (83)
Van Hare et al (121)	1996	10	12 ± 6	5.5 ± 3.8	2.1 ± 0.9	9/10 (90)
Baker et al (122)	1996	14	34 ± 25	> 0.5	3.3 ± 1.8	12/14 (86)
Triedman et al (123)	1995	10	23 ± 12	6.0 ± 5.4	3.6 ± 1.7	8/10 (80)
Lesh et al (55)	1994	6	20 ± 11	8.8 ± 7.4	3.5 ± 1.4	5/6 (83)

heart disease was repair of an atrial septal defect in 15 patients, transposition of the great arteries in 18 patients (Mustard procedure in 10, Senning procedure in 7, Rastelli procedure in 1), Fontan procedure for tricuspid atresia in 7, for double inlet single ventricle in 5 and for complex anomalies in 3 patients, and miscellaneous causes or types of surgery in another 10 patients. Incisional intraatrial reentrant tachycardias are usually sustained atrial arrhythmias with a constant atrial cycle length of more than 200 milliseconds, with sudden onset and termination of the tachycardia, an abnormal P wave morphology, and episodic Mobitz type I AV block without interruption of the primary tachycardia.

2. Electrophysiologic Characteristics and Diagnosis

A sustained atrial tachycardia occurring years after complex surgery for congenital heart disease is very suggestive of incisional reentry as an underlying mechanism. In the electrophysiology laboratory, entrainment techniques are applied in order to prove reentry as the underlying mechanism and characterize the anatomic barriers of the reentrant circuit.[37,55,121-123] *Manifest entrainment* is observed during a macroreentrant tachycardia if pacing is performed outside from the reentrant circuit (see Fig. 2); the surface ECG demonstrates constant fusion and the interval after termination of constant pacing is longer than 20 milliseconds. However, if pacing within the reentrant circuit is performed, *concealed entrainment* can usually be demonstrated; the P wave on the surface ECG is identical during pacing and during spontaneous tachycardia, stimulation artifact to surface P wave is equal to local electrogram to P wave, and the postpacing interval equals the tachycardia cycle length ± 10 milliseconds.[20,21] As in typical atrial flutter, concealed entrainment is observed in the isthmus that is considered critical for maintenance of the reentrant atrial tachycardia. A narrow isthmus of conduction, between a surgical scar and an anatomic barrier, for example, is the target for radiofrequency ablation. Additional techniques of mapping of incisional reentrant atrial tachycardias consist of the following: 1) search for split potentials, which are observed along conduction barriers and may represent surgical suture lines,[124] and 2) search for electrically silent areas, which may represent either scar or conduit or patch material.[37,101]

Despite the application of traditional mapping and entrainment techniques for radiofrequency catheter ablation of incisional reentrant tachycardias, the complexity of underlying congenital heart disease and multiple cardiac surgeries remains a considerable challenge. Individual surgical techniques and insufficient imaging modalities, usually based on biplane fluoroscopy, increase the challenge. Electroanatomic mapping[95–97,99,101] may be able to overcome some of the limitations of standard techniques. The electroanatomic, nonfluoroscopic mapping technique permits direct association of electrical activity with the underlying anatomic structures to identify the reentrant substrate and to target radiofrequency energy application more effectively (see Section IV). In addition, the ability to record and display features such as silent areas, based on visualization of low-voltage areas, and the ability to display lines of block, based on the delineation of double potentials, provides important adjunctive information to electrical activation display.

3. Therapy

The successful management of intraatrial reentrant tachycardia in patients who have undergone corrective surgery for congenital heart disease can be challenging. As demonstrated in Table 7, antiarrhythmic drugs, including most Class I drugs, are frequently ineffective. Class III antiarrhythmic drugs, especially amiodarone, may be more effective in some patients. In addition, antiarrhythmic agents have the potential to adversely affect myocardial function and exacerbate coexisting sinus node dysfunction; they may also have proarrhythmic effects. In severely symptomatic patients with continuous tachycardia, which puts the patient at an additional risk for a tachycardia-mediated cardiomyopathy, radiofrequency ablation of the AV junction and pacemaker implantation may be considered. However, the importance of the physiologic rate response in these patients may be considerable, and a pacemaker implantation can be an additional challenge depending on the underlying anatomy.

Radiofrequency catheter ablation in a critical isthmus of conduction, bounded by anatomic barriers, has therefore been attempted and was shown to be initially successful in 80% to 90% of patients (Table 7). Delineation of the critical isthmus with use of activation and entrainment mapping with several multielectrode catheters has been found to be critical for successful ablation. An example of a challenging patient is shown in Figures 25 through 27. Patient 8 is a 26-year-old female with a 4-year history of recurrent palpitations associated with dizziness and presyncope. Figure 25A shows the 12-lead ECG. Atypical P waves, predominantly negative in the inferior leads and in V_6, are present, with irregular AV conduction. The

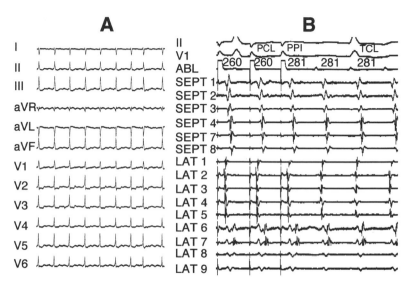

Figure 25. Twelve-lead ECG (A) and endocardial recordings (B) during atrial tachycardia in patient 8 with incisional intraatrial reentrant tachycardia. A. Atypical P waves with irregular atrioventricular conduction during atrial tachycardia are observed on the surface ECG. B. Entrainment mapping during intraatrial reentrant tachycardia. Pacing is performed with the ablation catheter (ABL) in the narrow isthmus between septal patch and tricuspid annulus patch. Endocardial recording is performed from a multipolar catheter positioned along the septum (SEPT 1–8) and along the lateral atrial free wall (LAT 1–9). The pacing cycle length (PCL) is 260 milliseconds, the tachycardia cycle length (TCL) is 281 milliseconds. After termination of pacing, the first atrial interval (postpacing interval [PPI]) is identical to the tachycardia cycle length (281 milliseconds) and the activation sequence and surface P wave morphology are the same. Thus, entrainment with concealed fusion from the isthmus between septal patch and tricuspid annulus patch suggests that pacing has been performed from an isthmus critical for maintaining reentrant excitation.

patient had a diagnosis of double-inlet left ventricle with transposition of the great arteries, and subsequently underwent placement of a Blalock-Taussig shunt. At the age of 13 years, she underwent a palliative Fontan procedure with oversewing of the tricuspid valve, patch closure of the atrial septal defect, and placement of a conduit between the right atrium and the pulmonary artery. Figure 26 shows a nonfluoroscopic electroanatomic map of the patient's reentrant atrial tachycardia. The gray regions represent electrically silent areas and demonstrate the pulmonary artery conduit, the patch closing the tricuspid annulus, and the septal patch. The color-coded isochronal map represents local activation times during atrial tachycardia, with red being early and blue-purple being late, based on an arbitrary temporal reference. In Figure 27, the electroanatomic map is displayed differently, such that activation can be traced during a cycle of reentry. In this activation map, the activation wavefront can be followed from the high right atrium, down between the pulmonary artery conduit and tricuspid annulus patch, turning around the tricuspid annulus patch, and coming up again between septal patch and tricuspid annulus patch. In this patient, the narrowest isthmus was found between the tricuspid annulus patch and the septal patch. Activation mapping in itself, however, cannot discern if a narrow isthmus is critical for maintenance of the reentrant tachycardia. If entrainment with manifest fusion is observed during pacing from such a potential isthmus, it is likely that pacing has been performed from outside the circuit, possibly representing an outer loop site. Thus, even though there is an isthmus, it may be an "innocent bystander." If entrainment with concealed fusion is present with the postponing interval after termination of pacing

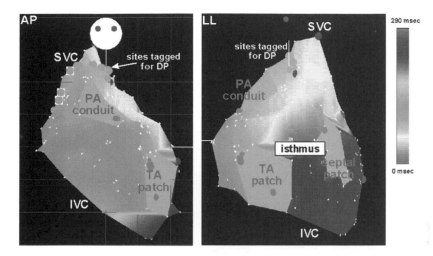

Figure 26. Anterior-posterior (AP) and left lateral (LL) view of a non-fluoroscopic electroanatomic mapping of an incisional intraatrial reentrant tachycardia in patient 8. Surgical barriers following the Fontan palliation, such as pulmonary artery (PA) conduit, tricuspid annulus (TA) patch, and septal (SEPT) patch, have been delineated during mapping based on very low or absent voltage from these regions. The probable site of a high right atrial surgical incision resulted in endocardial double potentials (DP), which are marked as pink dots. Interestingly, while this incision is present, it is not one of the critical barriers that delineate the reentry circuit in this case. The endocardial activation is represented using color-coded isochronal activation mapping with red earliest and purple latest. The activation map suggests a macroreentrant atrial tachycardia with a protected isthmus between TA patch and septal patch. IVC = inferior vena cava; SVC = superior vena cava. See color plate.

nearly equal to the spontaneous tachycardia cycle length (Fig. 25B), it is likely that the pacing site is within the critical tachycardia isthmus. That was the case in this patient, and successful ablation resulted from ablating along a line from the tricuspid annulus patch to the septal patch.

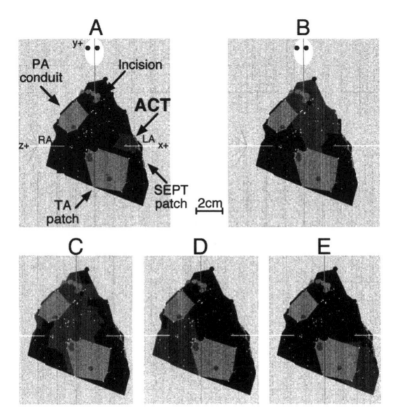

Figure 27. Activation mapping in patient 8 (same patient as in Figs. 24 and 25). A slightly left anterior oblique view of the activation map during different time intervals is shown, while the narrowing of the color range during activation allows consecutive images of the course of the activation wavefront (ACT). In the first image, the activation (light gray) starts superior to the septal patch (A), proceeds to the high atrium on both sides of the atrial incision (B), then enters a relatively wide isthmus between pulmonary artery conduit and tricuspid annulus patch (C), and travels around the tricuspid annulus patch (D) before it enters the narrow isthmus between tricuspid annulus and septal patch (E).

VII. Inappropriate Sinus Tachycardia

Inappropriate sinus tachycardia is an uncommon disorder. The underlying mechanism is still unclear and at present no rigorous diagnostic criteria for this syndrome exist. Previous studies[33,125,126] have suggested the presence of inappropriate sinus tachycardia if the following conditions are present: 1) a resting heart rate greater than 100 bpm or a heart rate increase to greater than 100 bpm with minimal exertion and a P wave morphology during tachycardia of sinus origin; 2) the correlation of symptoms with documented tachycardia; 3) the exclusion of secondary causes; and 4) the exclusion of a focal right atrial tachycardia (Table 8).

The pathophysiology of inappropriate sinus tachy-

Table 8

Diagnosis of Inappropriate Sinus Tachycardia

1) Documentation of tachycardia
   • Resting heart rate (supine/erect)
   • 24-hour Holter monitoring
   • Exercise stress test
2) Clear correlation of symptoms with tachycardia
3) Exclusion of secondary causes
   • Physical deconditioning
   • Orthostatic hypotension
   • Cardiac failure
   • Drug therapy
   • Endocrine and metabolic disorders
   • Anemia
4) Electrophysiologic testing
   • Exclusion of atrial tachycardia

cardia is still poorly understood, and differences between studies suggest a heterogeneous underlying condition. Abnormal autonomic influence on the sinus node, either excessive sympathetic tone or reduced vagal tone, is one possible explanation.[127] Another study found a normal autonomic balance in patients with inappropriate sinus tachycardia, but a significantly elevated intrinsic heart rate as well as β-adrenergic hypersensitivity and a depressed efferent cardiovagal reflex.[125] The authors conclude that a primary abnormality of sinus node function is present, manifest as enhanced automaticity.

1. Clinical and Electrocardiographic Presentation

Almost all patients with the clinical syndrome of inappropriate sinus tachycardia are young women; their mean age is approximately 30 years. Furthermore, many patients are health care professionals, especially nurses, and often cardiac or intensive care nurses. It is still unknown whether this striking observation is due to an unidentified occupational exposure, or if the syndrome in fact is more common but only recognized by persons who have access to sophisticated monitoring techniques. A recent preliminary study compared the psychiatric profile of patients with AV nodal reentrant tachycardia with that of those with inappropriate sinus tachycardia.[128] Patients with inappropriate sinus tachycardia were found to have symptom-amplification profiles that were also seen in patients with hypochondriasis, although there was otherwise no general indication of psychiatric disease.

Patients with the syndrome of inappropriate sinus tachycardia usually complain of frequent episodes of palpitations, dizziness, shortness of breath, and occasionally syncope. Furthermore, a reduction in exercise tolerance is frequently reported, with the symptoms ranging from intermittent to constant and incapacitating.

2. Electrophysiologic Characteristics and Diagnosis

The diagnosis of the syndrome of inappropriate sinus tachycardia is a clinical one that cannot be made solely on the basis of an electrophysiologic study. A stepwise approach toward the diagnosis of inappropriate sinus tachycardia is summarized in Table 8. The main goal of an electrophysiologic study is to exclude a sustained or nonsustained supraventricular tachycardia—atrial tachycardia in particular. Furthermore, heart rate and site of earliest crista terminalis activation can be determined during sympathetic stimulation and vagal maneuvers. It has been demonstrated that the sinus node pacemaker complex is distributed along the long axis of the crista terminalis, extending from the junction of the superior vena cava with the right atrium almost down to the junction of the inferior vena cava.[30,31] Furthermore, sinus node tissue may also be found in the superior and medial extent of the crista terminalis as it crosses anterior to the superior vena cava.[30,33] In order to map the crista terminalis, a deflectable multipolar catheter is advanced into the right atrium via a long vascular sheath to ensure stability (see Fig. 30). Intracardiac ultrasound is used to confirm the position of the multipolar catheter along the crista. Subsequently, heart rate and earliest activation along the crista terminalis are noted.

Patients with inappropriate sinus tachycardia have

been found to have an increased sensitivity to isoproterenol.[127] Furthermore, there is a progressive superior shift in the site of earliest activation along the crista during isoproterenol infusion, associated with an increase in heart rate, as well as an inferior shift during vagal maneuvers, associated with a decrease in heart rate.[33] The increase or decrease is always gradual, as compared to a warm up and cool down phenomenon during focal (ectopic) tachycardia, which usually lasts only 3 to 5 beats (see Fig. 13). It is crucial to distinguish between automatic atrial tachycardia and inappropriate sinus, as medical and ablative therapies differ. Compared to the shift of early activation of sinus tachycardia during isoproterenol infusion, the earliest site of activation during atrial tachycardia remains fixed, even though the rate may change as a result of alteration in autonomic tone. In addition, the appearance of the local electrogram during atrial tachycardia is fractionated and early (>30 milliseconds with respect to P wave onset; see Fig. 13), whereas during sinus tachycardia, it generally has a normal configuration.

3. Therapy

As no comparative studies of the management of inappropriate sinus tachycardia exist, the therapeutic approaches are empirical. The first-line therapy should be pharmacological; the agents most frequently used are β-blockers and calcium channel blockers. Class Ia or Ic drugs may be effective in some patients. Although amiodarone may suppress sinus node function, the risk-benefit ratio is unknown, as it might mean long-term treatment in young patients with a non-life-threatening condition.

The decision regarding which patient should

undergo an invasive procedure, such as sinus node modification, sinus node ablation, or ablation of the AV junction with subsequent pacemaker implantation, is based on the duration of symptoms, the failure of reasonably exhaustive medical therapy, the exclusion of other tachycardias and reversible conditions, and an extensive discussion with the patient about the benefits and risks. Some patients complain of symptoms not in relation to a documented tachycardia, such as fatigue, lack of drive, or depression. Patients must understand that only those symptoms clearly associated with a rapid heart rate can improve with sinus node ablation.

Figure 28 shows a continuous ECG recording dur-

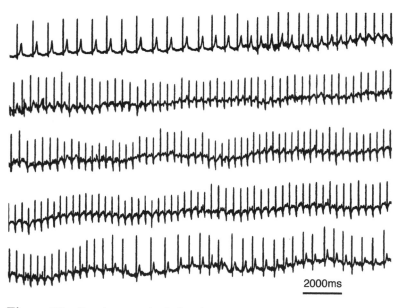

2000ms

Figure 28. Continuous single-lead ECG recording during Holter monitoring in patient 9, who has the syndrome of inappropriate sinus tachycardia. Note the gradual increase and decrease in heart rate, following mild exercise.

ing Holter monitoring from patient 9, a 33-year-old female nurse. The patient complained of frequent episodes of palpitations associated with exhaustion even after mild exercise such that the patient was no longer able to follow her personal or professional interests. As characteristically observed, the resting heart rate was high-normal at 85 bpm and increased to 165 bpm during what was reported as minimal exercise. Both the onset and termination of the increased heart rate were gradual. Figure 29 shows the heart rate trend over 24 hours. A high-normal resting heart rate of approximately 80 bpm was interrupted by frequent episodes of tachycardia up to a rate of 170 bpm, again during reported minimal exercise.

The current approach to sinus node modification in

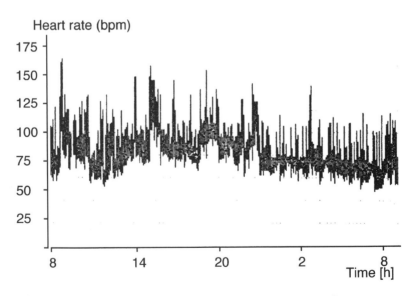

Figure 29. Twenty-four-hour heart rate trend during Holter monitoring in patient 9, who has inappropriate sinus tachycardia.

our electrophysiologic laboratory is a combined anatomic and electrophysiologic approach.[32,33] Mapping of the crista terminalis is performed as described. During isoproterenol infusion, an increase in heart rate and a cranial shift of the sinus node pacemaker is observed. After identification of the site of earliest activation along a catheter placed on the crista terminalis, mapping is performed with the ablation catheter. The proximity of the tip of the ablation catheter to the crista terminalis is confirmed with intracardiac ultrasound (Fig. 30). Radiofrequency energy is applied during isoproterenol infusion, usually starting in the high lateral right atrium, close to the junction with the superior vena cava. Radiofrequency applications are then targeted sequentially to progressively inferior sites along the crista terminalis as the sinus node function is shifted inferiorly with successful sinus node modification. In Figure 31, a progressive inferior shift of sinus node pacemaker function can be observed during radiofrequency application, associated with a significant reduction in heart rate.

In a series of 28 patients, an acutely successful sinus node modification was achieved in 21 patients (75%), defined as an increase in sinus cycle length of at least 10% on matched doses of isoproterenol and atropine.[33,129] Concomitantly, a marked inferior shift in the surface ECG P wave axis was documented, consistent with the progressively inferior shift of the sinus node pacemaker function following successful sinus node modification. However, the high early electrophysiologic success rate is tempered by a high recurrence rate[130]: only 40% of the patients had sustained improvement of tachycardia symptoms 8 ± 5 months after sinus node modification, whereas a repeat ablation was required in 32% of these patients. In case of recurrence, a more aggressive ablation

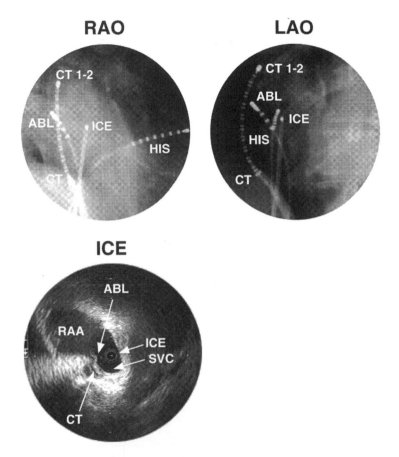

Figure 30. Fluoroscopic right anterior oblique (RAO) and left anterior oblique (LAO) catheter position, as well as intracardiac echocardiographic imaging (ICE) during mapping and ablation of inappropriate sinus tachycardia. A 20-pole catheter is placed along the crista terminalis (CT; tip CT 1–2) using a long vascular sheath. An octopolar catheter is positioned along the septum (HIS). The tip of the ablation catheter (ABL) is in the area of the high crista terminalis. The ICE is a cross section at the junction between superior vena cava and right atrium. The right atrial appendage (RAA) is seen just opening at this level. The tip of the ablation catheter with the characteristic fan shape is located right on the crista terminalis along the high anterolateral right atrium.

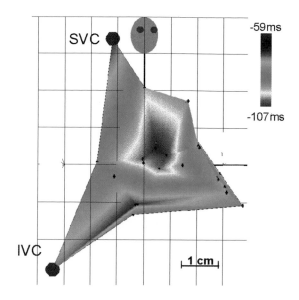

Figure 16.

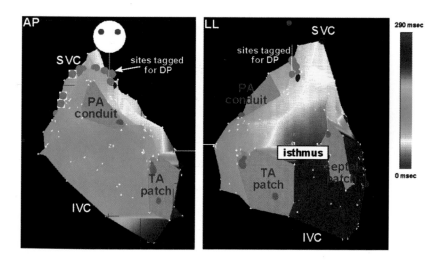

Figure 26.

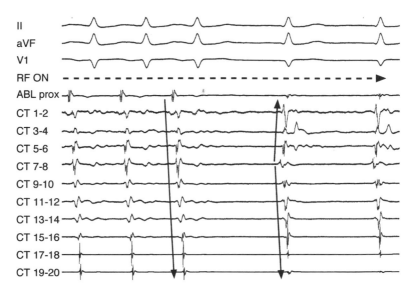

Figure 31. Surface and endocardial recording during ablation of inappropriate sinus tachycardia with the catheters in position as shown in Figure 29. During radiofrequency application (RF ON), after the third beat, a sudden decrease in rate is observed. Furthermore, a shift of the site of earliest activation from the high crista (bipole 3–4 on the CT catheter) to the mid crista terminalis is observed (bipole 7–8).

attempt can be performed, including attempts at total ablation of sinus node function with permanent pacemaker implantation.

VIII. Conclusion

In the last several years, "atrial arrhythmology" has emerged as a topic of great interest within the electrophysiologic community. Our knowledge of tachycardia mechanism has expanded greatly, as new information has been revealed during electrophysiologic assessment in patients both with and without structural heart disease. What has become clear is that the term "atrial tachycardia" is a broad one, which includes a number of separate and distinct subtypes. The recognition of distinct subsets has in turn led to the development of catheter-based ablative approaches which are specific to the mechanism of the atrial tachycardia in question.

Thus, "automatic" or "focal" ectopic atrial tachycardia can be mapped and ablated in a small region identified as the site of early activation. On the other hand, macroreentrant atrial tachycardia, such as that which occurs in patients with prior surgical repair of congenital heart disease, requires an ablative approach that targets a critical isthmus. Patients with the syndrome of inappropriate sinus tachycardia require progressive ablation along the crista terminalis in order to modify sinus node function.

It is also of interest that atrial tachycardias are not randomly distributed, but tend to occur at certain locations in the atrium, consistent with the hypothesis that atrial anatomy is the primary determinant of atrial electrophysiologic function and arrhythmogenesis. Finally, and perhaps most importantly, we now recognize that many cases of atrial fibrillation may be initiated by focal firing. If the astounding observation that the pulmonary veins are the site of origin for the vast majority of these atrial fibrillation triggers is confirmed, we may well be within striking distance of a catheter-based cure for this most common of all atrial arrhythmias.

References

1. Lesh MD, Kalman JM. To fumble flutter or tackle "tach"? Toward updated classifiers for atrial tachy-

arrhythmias. *J Cardiovasc Electrophysiol* 1996;7: 460–466.

2. Lesh MD, Kalman JM, Karch MR. Use of intracardiac echocardiography during electrophysiologic evaluation and therapy of atrial arrhythmias. *J Cardiovasc Electrophysiol* 1998;9:S40-S47.

3. Chu E, Kalman JM, Kwasman MA, et al. Intracardiac echocardiography during radiofrequency catheter ablation of cardiac arrhythmias in humans. *J Am Coll Cardiol* 1994;24:1351–1357.

4. Chu E, Fitzpatrick AP, Chin MC, et al. Radiofrequency catheter ablation guided by intracardiac echocardiography. *Circulation* 1994;89:1301–1305.

5. SippensGroenewegen A, Peeters HA, Jessurun ER, et al. Body surface mapping during pacing at multiple sites in the human atrium: P-wave morphology of ectopic right atrial activation. *Circulation* 1998;97: 369–380.

6. SippensGroenewegen A, Roithinger FX, Scholtz DB, et al. Noninvasive localization or right atrial tachycardia using an atlas of paced P wave body surface integral map patterns. *Pacing Clin Electrophysiol* 1998;21:858.

7. SippensGroenewegen A, Roithinger FX, Mlynash MD, et al. 62-lead ECG map—analysis of T wave obscured ectopic atrial beats using automated QRST subtraction. *Circulation* 1998;98:I-25. Abstract.

8. Scheinman MM, Basu D, Hollenberg M. Electrophysiologic studies in patients with persistent atrial tachycardia. *Circulation* 1974;50:266–273.

9. Gillette PC, Garson A Jr. Electrophysiologic and pharmacologic characteristics of automatic ectopic atrial tachycardia. *Circulation* 1977;56:571–575.

10. Coumel P, Flammang D, Attuel P, Leclercq JF. Sus-

tained intra-atrial reentrant tachycardia. Electrophysiologic study of 20 cases. *Clin Cardiol* 1979;2: 167–178.

11. Wu D, Amat-y-Leon F, Denes P, et al. Demonstration of sustained sinus and atrial re-entry as a mechanism of paroxysmal supraventricular tachycardia. *Circulation* 1975;51:234–243.

12. Akhtar M, Jazayeri MR, Sra J, et al. Atrioventricular nodal reentry. Clinical, electrophysiological, and therapeutic considerations. *Circulation* 1993;88: 282–295.

13. Jackman WM, Beckman KJ, McClelland JH, et al. Treatment of supraventricular tachycardia due to atrioventricular nodal reentry, by radiofrequency catheter ablation of slow-pathway conduction. *N Engl J Med* 1992;327:313–318.

14. Lee MA, Morady F, Kadish A, et al. Catheter modification of the atrioventricular junction with radiofrequency energy for control of atrioventricular nodal reentry tachycardia. *Circulation* 1991;83:827–835.

15. Ruder MA, Davis JC, Eldar M, et al. Clinical and electrophysiologic characterization of automatic junctional tachycardia in adults. *Circulation* 1986;73: 930–937.

16. Scheinman MM, Gonzalez RP, Cooper MW, et al. Clinical and electrophysiologic features and role of catheter ablation techniques in adult patients with automatic atrioventricular junctional tachycardia. *Am J Cardiol* 1994;74:565–572.

17. Hamdan M, Van Hare GF, Fisher W, et al. Selective catheter ablation of the tachycardia focus in patients with nonreentrant junctional tachycardia. *Am J Cardiol* 1996;78:1292–1297.

18. Jackman WM, Wang XZ, Friday KJ, et al. Catheter

ablation of accessory atrioventricular pathways (Wolff-Parkinson-White syndrome) by radiofrequency current. *N Engl J Med* 1991;324:1605–1611.

19. Lesh MD, Van Hare GF, Schamp DJ, et al. Curative percutaneous catheter ablation using radiofrequency energy for accessory pathways in all locations: Results in 100 consecutive patients. *J Am Coll Cardiol* 1992;19:1303–1309.

20. Olgin JE, Kalman JM, Fitzpatrick AP, Lesh MD. Role of right atrial endocardial structures as barriers to conduction during human type I atrial flutter. Activation and entrainment mapping guided by intracardiac echocardiography. *Circulation* 1995;92: 1839–1848.

21. Kalman JM, Olgin JE, Saxon LA, et al. Activation and entrainment mapping defines the tricuspid annulus as the anterior barrier in typical atrial flutter. *Circulation* 1996;94:398–406.

22. Nakagawa H, Lazzara R, Khastgir T, et al. Role of the tricuspid annulus and the eustachian valve/ridge on atrial flutter. Relevance to catheter ablation of the septal isthmus and a new technique for rapid identification of ablation success. *Circulation* 1996;94: 407–424.

23. Saxon LA, Kalman JM, Olgin JE, et al. Results of radiofrequency catheter ablation for atrial flutter. *Am J Cardiol* 1996;77:1014–1016.

24. Tai CT, Chen SA, Chiang CE, et al. Long-term outcome of radiofrequency catheter ablation for typical atrial flutter: Risk prediction of recurrent arrhythmias. *J Cardiovasc Electrophysiol* 1998;9:115–121.

25. Kalman JM, Olgin JE, Saxon LA, et al Electrocardiographic and electrophysiologic characterization of atypical atrial flutter in man: Use of activation and

entrainment mapping and implications for catheter ablation. *J Cardiovasc Electrophysiol* 1997;8: 121–144.

26. Narula OS. Sinus node re-entry: A mechanism for supraventricular tachycardia. *Circulation* 1974;50: 1114–1128.

27. Gomes JA, Hariman RJ, Kang PS, Chowdry IH. Sustained symptomatic sinus node reentrant tachycardia: Incidence, clinical significance, electrophysiologic observations and the effects of antiarrhythmic agents. *J Am Coll Cardiol* 1985;5:45–57.

28. Kerr CR, Klein GG, Guiraudon GM, Webb JG. Surgical therapy for sinoatrial reentrant tachycardia. *Pacing Clin Electrophysiol* 1988;11:776–783.

29. Sanders WE Jr, Sorrentino RA, Greenfield RA, et al. Catheter ablation of sinoatrial node reentrant tachycardia. *J Am Coll Cardiol* 1994;23:926–934.

30. Anderson KR, Ho SY, Anderson RH. Location and vascular supply of sinus node in human heart. *Br Heart J* 1979;41:28–32.

31. Boineau JP, Canavan TE, Schuessler RB, et al. Demonstration of a widely distributed atrial pacemaker complex in the human heart. *Circulation* 1988;77: 1221–1237.

32. Kalman JM, Lee RJ, Fisher WG, et al. Radiofrequency catheter modification of sinus pacemaker function guided by intracardiac echocardiography. *Circulation* 1995;92:3070–3081.

33. Lee RJ, Kalman JM, Fitzpatrick AP, et al. Radiofrequency catheter modification of the sinus node for "inappropriate" sinus tachycardia. *Circulation* 1995;92:2919–2928.

34. Wellens HJ. Atrial tachycardia. How important is the mechanism? *Circulation* 1994;90:1576–1577.

35. Chen SA, Chiang CE, Yang CJ, et al. Sustained atrial tachycardia in adult patients. Electrophysiological characteristics, pharmacological response, possible mechanisms, and effects of radiofrequency ablation. *Circulation* 1994;90:1262−1278.

36. Engelstein ED, Lippman N, Stein KM, Lerman BB. Mechanism-specific effects of adenosine on atrial tachycardia. *Circulation* 1994;89:2645−2654.

37. Kalman JM, VanHare GF, Olgin JE, et al. Ablation of 'incisional' reentrant atrial tachycardia complicating surgery for congenital heart disease. Use of entrainment to define a critical isthmus of conduction. *Circulation* 1996;93:502−512.

38. Lesh MD, Kalman JM, Saxon LA, Dorostkar PC. Electrophysiology of "incisional" reentrant atrial tachycardia complicating surgery for congenital heart disease. *Pacing Clin Electrophysiol* 1997;20: 2107−2111.

39. Lesh MD, Kalman JM, Olgin JE, Ellis WS. The role of atrial anatomy in clinical atrial arrhythmias. *J Electrocardiol* 1996;29(suppl):101−113.

40. Spach MS, Dolber PC, Heidlage JF. Influence of the passive anisotropic properties on directional differences in propagation following modification of the sodium conductance in human atrial muscle. A model of reentry based on anisotropic discontinuous propagation. *Circ Res* 1988;62:811−832.

41. Spach MS, Josephson ME. Initiating reentry: The role of nonuniform anisotropy in small circuits. *J Cardiovasc Electrophysiol* 1994;5:182−209.

42. Saffitz JE, Kanter HL, Green KG, et al. Tissue-specific determinants of anisotropic conduction velocity in canine atrial and ventricular myocardium. *Circ Res* 1994;74:1065−1070.

43. Spach MS, Miller WTd, Geselowitz DB, et al. The discontinuous nature of propagation in normal canine cardiac muscle. Evidence for recurrent discontinuities of intracellular resistance that affect the membrane currents. *Circ Res* 1981;48:39–54.
44. Chen SA, Tai CT, Chiang CE, et al. Focal atrial tachycardia: Reanalysis of the clinical and electrophysiologic characteristics and prediction of successful radiofrequency ablation. *J Cardiovasc Electrophysiol* 1998;9:355–365.
45. Josephson M. Supraventricular tachycardia. In Josephson M (ed): *Clinical Cardiac Electrophysiology.* Malvern, PA: Lea & Febiger; 1993:256–265.
46. Chen SA, Chiang CE, Yang CJ, et al. Radiofrequency catheter ablation of sustained intra-atrial reentrant tachycardia in adult patients. Identification of electrophysiological characteristics and endocardial mapping techniques. *Circulation* 1993;88:578–587.
47. Gillette PC, Crawford FC, Zeiger VL. Mechanisms of atrial tachycardia. In Zipes DP, Jalife J (eds): *Cardiac Electrophysiology: From Cell to Bedside.* Philadelphia, PA: Saunders Publishing Co.; 1990:559–563.
48. Garson A, Smith RT, Moak JP, et al. Atrial automatic ectopic tachycardia in children. In Touboul P, Waldo AL (eds): *Atrial Arrhythmias: Current Concepts and Management.* St. Louis, MO: Mosby Yearbook; 1990:282–287.
49. Joyner RW, van Capelle FJ. Propagation through electrically coupled cells. How a small SA node drives a large atrium. *Biophys J* 1986;50:1157–1164.
50. Kalman JM, Olgin JE, Karch MR, et al. "Cristal tachycardias": Origin of right atrial tachycardias from the crista terminalis identified by intracardiac echocardiography. *J Am Coll Cardiol* 1998;31:451–459.

51. Pappone C, Stabile G, De Simone A, et al. Role of catheter-induced mechanical trauma in localization of target sites of radiofrequency ablation in automatic atrial tachycardia. *J Am Coll Cardiol* 1996;27: 1090–1097.

52. Poty H, Saoudi N, Hassaguerre M, et al. Radiofrequency catheter ablation of atrial tachycardias. *Am Heart J* 1996;131:481–489.

53. Tang CW, Scheinman MM, Van Hare GF, et al. Use of P wave configuration during atrial tachycardia to predict site of origin. *J Am Coll Cardiol* 1995;26: 1315–1324.

54. Feld GK. Catheter ablation for the treatment of atrial tachycardia. *Prog Cardiovasc Dis* 1995;37:205–224.

55. Lesh MD, Van Hare GF, Epstein LM, et al. Radiofrequency catheter ablation of atrial arrhythmias. Results and mechanisms. *Circulation* 1994;89: 1074–1089.

56. Goldberger J, Kall J, Ehlert F, et al. Effectiveness of radiofrequency catheter ablation for treatment of atrial tachycardia. *Am J Cardiol* 1993;72:787–793.

57. Kay GN, Chong F, Epstein AE, et al. Radiofrequency ablation for treatment of primary atrial tachycardias. *J Am Coll Cardiol* 1993;21:901–909.

58. Tracy CM, Swartz JF, Fletcher RD, et al. Radiofrequency catheter ablation of ectopic atrial tachycardia using paced activation sequence mapping. *J Am Coll Cardiol* 1993;21:910–917.

59. Walsh EP, Saul JP, Hulse JE, et al. Transcatheter ablation of ectopic atrial tachycardia in young patients using radiofrequency current. *Circulation* 1992;86: 1138–1146.

60. Gillette PC, Wampler DG, Garson A Jr, et al. Treat-

ment of atrial automatic tachycardia by ablation procedures. *J Am Coll Cardiol* 1985;6:405–409.

61. Wyndham CR, Arnsdorf MF, Levitsky S, et al. Successful surgical excision of focal paroxysmal atrial tachycardia. Observations in vivo and in vitro. *Circulation* 1980;62:1365–1372.

62. Johnson NJ, Rosen MR. The distinction between triggered activity and other cardiac arrhythmias. In Brugada P, Wellens HJJ (eds): *Cardiac Arrhythmias: Where to Go From Here?* Mt. Kisco, NY: Futura Publishing Co., 1987:129–145.

63. Rosen M. Cellular electrophysiology of digitalis toxicity. *J Am Coll Cardiol* 1985;5:22–34.

64. Ferrier G. Digitalis arrhythmias: Role of oscillatory afterpotentials. *Prog Cardiovasc Dis* 1977;19: 459–474.

65. Kojima M, Sperelakis N. Effects of calcium channel blockers on ouabain-induced oscillatory afterpotentials in organ-cultured young embryonic chick hearts. *Eur J Pharmacol* 1986;122:65–73.

66. Man KC, Chan KK, Kovack P, et al. Spatial resolution of atrial pace mapping as determined by unipolar atrial pacing at adjacent sites. *Circulation* 1996;94: 1357–1363.

67. Gillette PC, Smith RT, Garson A Jr, et al. Chronic supraventricular tachycardia. A curable cause of congestive cardiomyopathy. *JAMA* 1985;253: 391–392.

68. Gillette PC. Supraventricular arrhythmias in children. *J Am Coll Cardiol* 1985;5:122B–129B.

69. Packer DL, Bardy GH, Worley SJ, et al. Tachycardia-induced cardiomyopathy: A reversible form of left ventricular dysfunction. *Am J Cardiol* 1986;57: 563–570.

70. Ott DA, Gillette PC, Garson A Jr. Surgical management of refractory supraventricular tachycardia in infants and children. *J Am Coll Cardiol* 1985;5: 124–129.

71. Shine KI, Kastor JA, Yurchak PM. Multifocal atrial tachycardia. Clinical and electrocardiographic features in 32 patients. *N Engl J Med* 1968;279:344–349.

72. Lipson MJ, Naimi S. Multifocal atrial tachycardia (chaotic atrial tachycardia). Clinical associations and significance. *Circulation* 1970;42:397–407.

73. Phillips J, Spano J, Burch G. Chaotic atrial mechanism. *Am Heart J* 1969;78:171–179.

74. Scher D, Arsura E. Multifocal atrial tachycardia: Mechanisms, clinical correlates and treatment. *Am Heart J* 1989;118:574–580.

75. Lin C, Chuang I, Chenk K, Chiang B. Arrhythmogenic effects of theophylline in human atrial tissue. *Int J Cardiol* 1987;17:289–297.

76. Levine J, Michael J, Guarnieri T. Multifocal atrial tachycardia: A toxic effect of theophylline. *Lancet* 1985;1(8419):12–14.

77. Kastor J. Multifocal atrial tachycardia. *N Engl J Med* 1990;322:1713–1717.

78. Stock J. Beta adrenergic blocking drugs in the clinical management of cardiac arrhythmias. *Am J Cardiol* 1966;18:444–449.

79. Harrison D, Griffin J, Fiene T. Effects of beta-adrenergic blockade with propranolol in patients with atrial arrhythmias. *N Engl J Med* 1965;273:410–415.

80. Berns E, Rinkenberger RL, Jeang MK, et al. Efficacy and safety of flecainide acetate for atrial tachycardia or fibrillation. *Am J Cardiol* 1987;59:1337–1341.

81. Till JA, Rowland E, Shinebourne EA, Ward DE. Treatment of refractory supraventricular arrhyth-

mias with flecainide acetate. *Arch Dis Child* 1987;
62:247–252.
82. Coumel P, Leclercq J, Assayag P. European experience with the antiarrhythmic efficacy of propafenone for supraventricular arrhythmias. *Am J Cardiol*
1984;54:60–66.
83. Pool P, Quart B. Treatment of ectopic atrial arrhythmias and premature atrial complexes in adults with
encainide. *Am J Cardiol* 1988;62:60–62.
84. Brugada P, Abdollah H, Wellens H, Paulussen G.
Suppression of incessant supraventricular tachycardia by intravenous and oral encainide. *J Am Coll
Cardiol* 1984;4:1255–1260.
85. Haines DE, DiMarco JP. Sustained intraatrial reentrant tachycardia: Clinical, electrocardiographic and
electrophysiologic characteristics and long-term follow-up. *J Am Coll Cardiol* 1990;15:1345–1354.
86. Kopelman H, Horowitz L. Efficacy and toxicity of
amiodarone for the treatment of supraventricular
tachyarrhythmias. *Prog Cardiovasc Dis* 1989;31:
355–366.
87. Irons G, Ginn W, Orgain E. Use of a beta adrenergic
receptor blocking agent (propranolol) in the treatment of cardiac arrhythmias. *Am J Med* 1967;43:
161–170.
88. El-Sherif N. Supraventricular tachycardia with AV
block. *Br Heart J* 1970;32:46–56.
89. Bertil Olsson S, Blomstrom P, Sabel KG, William-
Olsson G. Incessant ectopic atrial tachycardia: Successful surgical treatment with regression of dilated
cardiomyopathy picture. *Am J Cardiol* 1984;53:
1465–1466.
90. Packer DB, Johnson SB. Intracardiac ultrasound

guidance of linear lesion creation for ablation of atrial fibrillation. *J Am Coll Cardiol* 1998;31:333A.
91. Roithinger FX, Steiner PR, Goseki Y, et al. A stepwise approach for creating linear lesions: Intracardiac echocardiography and low-power radiofrequency application. *Eur Heart J* 1998;19:537. Abstract.
92. Karch MR, Zrenner B, Weyerbrock S, et al. Intracardiac multielectrode mapping with the "basket" catheter demonstrates distinct activation patterns before termination of human atrial fibrillation. *Pacing Clin Electrophysiol* 1998;21:958. Abstract.
93. Zrenner B, Schneider MAE, Hofmann F, et al. Three-dimensional computer-assisted animation of atrial tachyarrhythmias recorded with a 64-polar basket catheter. *Eur Heart J* 1998;19:196. Abstract.
94. Schmitt C, Zrenner B, Schneider M, et al. Clinical experience with a novel multielectrode basket catheter in right atrial tachycardias. *Circulation* 1999;99: 2414–2422.
95. Shpun S, Gepstein L, Hayam G, Ben-Haim SA. Guidance of radiofrequency endocardial ablation with real-time three-dimensional magnetic navigation system. *Circulation* 1997;96:2016–2021.
96. Gepstein L, Hayam G, Ben-Haim SA. A novel method for nonfluoroscopic catheter-based electroanatomical mapping of the heart. In vitro and in vivo accuracy results. *Circulation* 1997;95:1611–1622.
97. Gepstein L, Ben-Haim SA. 3D cardiac imaging of electromechanical coupling. *Adv Exp Med Biol* 1997;430:303–311.
98. Shah DC, Jas P, Hassaguerre M, et al. Three-dimensional mapping of the common atrial flutter circuit in the right atrium. *Circulation* 1997;96:3904–3912.

99. Smeets JL, Ben-Haim SA, Rodriguez LM, et al. New method for nonfluoroscopic endocardial mapping in humans: Accuracy assessment and first clinical results. *Circulation* 1998;97:2426–2432.

100. Kottkamp H, Hindricks G, Breithardt G, Borggrefe M. Three-dimensional electromagnetic catheter technology: Electroanatomical mapping of the right atrium and ablation of ectopic atrial tachycardia. *J Cardiovasc Electrophysiol* 1997;8:1332–1337.

101. Dorostkar PC, Cheng J, Scheinman MM. Electroanatomic mapping and ablation of the substrate supporting intra-atrial reentrant tachycardia after palliation for complex congenital heart disease. *Pacing Clin Electrophysiol* 1999;21:1810–1819.

102. Schilling R, Peters N, Kadish A, Davies W. Characterization of human atrial flutter using a novel noncontact mapping system. *Pacing Clin Electrophysiol* 1997;20:1054. Abstract.

103. Schilling R, Peters N, Davies W. Results of radiofrequency catheter ablation of human left ventricular tachycardia guided by a non-contact mapping system. *Pacing Clin Electrophysiol* 1998;21:922. Abstract.

104. Kadish A, Schilling R, Peters N, et al. Endocardial mapping of human atrial fibrillation using a novel non-contact mapping system. *Pacing Clin Electrophysiol* 1997;20:1063.

105. Moe G. On the multiple wavelet hypothesis of atrial fibrillation. *Arch Int Pharmacodyn Ther* 1962;140:183.

106. Cox JL, Schuessler RB, D'Agostino HJ Jr, et al. The surgical treatment of atrial fibrillation. III. Development of a definitive surgical procedure. *J Thorac Cardiovasc Surg* 1991;101:569–583.

107. Cox JL, Boineau JP, Schuessler RB, et al. Five-year experience with the maze procedure for atrial fibrillation. *Ann Thorac Surg* 1993;56:814–824.

108. Hassaguerre M, Gencel L, Fischer B, et al. Successful catheter ablation of atrial fibrillation. *J Cardiovasc Electrophysiol* 1994;5:1045–1052.

109. Hassaguerre M, Jas P, Shah DC, et al. Right and left atrial radiofrequency catheter therapy of paroxysmal atrial fibrillation. *J Cardiovasc Electrophysiol* 1996; 7:1132–1144.

110. Jas P, Hassaguerre M, Shah DC, et al. A focal source of atrial fibrillation treated by discrete radiofrequency ablation. *Circulation* 1997;95:572–576.

111. Hassaguerre M, Jas P, Shah DC, et al. Spontaneous initiation of atrial fibrillation by ectopic beats originating in the pulmonary veins. *N Engl J Med* 1998; 339:659–666.

112. Wijffels MC, Kirchhof CJ, Dorland R, Allessie MA. Atrial fibrillation begets atrial fibrillation. A study in awake chronically instrumented goats. *Circulation* 1995;92:1954–1968.

113. Daoud EG, Bogun F, Goyal R, et al. Effect of atrial fibrillation on atrial refractoriness in humans. *Circulation* 1996;94:1600–1606.

114. Nathan H, Eliakim M. The junction between the left atrium and the pulmonary veins. An anatomic study of human hearts. *Circulation* 1966;34:412–422.

115. Lesh MD, Guerra P, Roithinger FX, et al. Novel technology for catheter ablative cure of atrial fibrillation. *J Intervent Electrophysiol* 1999. In press.

116. Spach MS, Barr RC, Jewett PH. Spread of excitation from the atrium into thoracic veins in human beings and dogs. *Am J Cardiol* 1972;30:844–854.

117. Satoh T, Zipes DP. Unequal atrial stretch in dogs

increases dispersion of refractoriness conducive to developing atrial fibrillation. *J Cardiovasc Electrophysiol* 1996;7:833–842.

118. Wijffels MC, Kirchhof CJ, Dorland R, et al. Electrical remodeling due to atrial fibrillation in chronically instrumented conscious goats: Roles of neurohumoral changes, ischemia, atrial stretch, and high rate of electrical activation. *Circulation* 1997;96: 3710–3720.

119. Ausma J, Wijffels M, Thone F, et al. Structural changes of atrial myocardium due to sustained atrial fibrillation in the goat. *Circulation* 1997;96: 3157–3163.

120. Flinn CJ, Wolff GS, Dick MD, et al. Cardiac rhythm after the Mustard operation for complete transposition of the great arteries. *N Engl J Med* 1984;310: 1635–1638.

121. Van Hare GF, Lesh MD, Ross BA, et al. Mapping and radiofrequency ablation of intraatrial reentrant tachycardia after the Senning or Mustard procedure for transposition of the great arteries. *Am J Cardiol* 1996;77:985–991.

122. Baker BM, Lindsay BD, Bromberg BI, et al. Catheter ablation of clinical intraatrial reentrant tachycardias resulting from previous atrial surgery: Localizing and transecting the critical isthmus. *J Am Coll Cardiol* 1996;28:411–417.

123. Triedman JK, Saul JP, Weindling SN, Walsh EP. Radiofrequency ablation of intra-atrial reentrant tachycardia after surgical palliation of congenital heart disease. *Circulation* 1995;91:707–714.

124. Olshansky B, Okumura K, Henthorn RW, Waldo AL. Characterization of double potentials in human

atrial flutter: Studies during transient entrainment. *J Am Coll Cardiol* 1990;15:833–841.

125. Morillo CA, Klein GJ, Thakur RK, et al. Mechanism of 'inappropriate' sinus tachycardia. Role of sympathovagal balance. *Circulation* 1994;90:873–877.

126. Krahn AD, Yee R, Klein GJ, Morillo C. Inappropriate sinus tachycardia: Evaluation and therapy. *J Cardiovasc Electrophysiol* 1995;6:1124–1128.

127. Bauernfeind RA, Amat-y-Leon F, Dhingra RC, et al. Chronic nonparoxysmal sinus tachycardia in otherwise healthy persons. *Ann Intern Med* 1979;91: 702–710.

128. Zivin A, Glick R, Knight BP, et al. Psychiatric profile of patients with inappropriate sinus tachycardia. *Pacing Clin Electrophysiol* 1998;21:923.

129. Shinbane JS, Lee RJ, Evans JT, et al. Electrophysiologic and electrocardiographic manifestations of transcatheter radiofrequency sinus node modification in humans. *Pacing Clin Electrophysiol* 1996;19: 594.

130. Shinbane JS, Lee R, Evans T, et al. Long-term follow-up after radiofrequency sinus node modification for inappropriate sinus tachycardia. *J Am Coll Cardiol* 1997;29:199A.

Index

Page numbers followed by *f* indicate figures.